What to Expect (*from God*) When You're Expecting

by Cathy Hickling

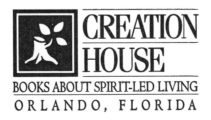

CREATION HOUSE

BOOKS ABOUT SPIRIT-LED LIVING

ORLANDO, FLORIDA

Creation House
Strang Communications Company
600 Rinehart Road
Lake Mary, FL 32746
(407) 333-3132
Fax: (407) 283-8494

Unless otherwise noted, Scripture quotations are from
the Holy Bible, New International Version.
Copyright © 1973, 1978, 1984, International Bible Society. Used by
permission.

Scripture quotations marked KJV are from
the King James Version of the Bible.

Scripture quotations marked NAS are from the New American Standard
Bible. Copyright © 1960, 1962, 1963, 1968, 1971, 1972, 1973, 1975,
1977 by the Lockman Foundation. Used by permission.

Scripture quotations marked NEB are from the
New English Bible. Copyright © 1961, 1970 by the Delegates of the
Oxford University Press and the
Syndics of the Cambridge University Press.
Used by permission.

Illustrations by Diane M. Vivian

Revised Edition:
First printing, July 1995
Second printing, August 1995
Third printing, September 1995

Dedication

*With love to my babies,
Holly, David, Benjamin and the one I'm carrying
as I write this book*

Acknowledgments

A pregnant woman is a needy woman. I acknowledge my need for the many people who made this book possible.

Thanks to my friends and family for your help, encouragement and support. God bless you, Dr. Edward Austin, Barb and the *Expression* staff, Katie and everyone at the Bethany Guest House. Thanks especially to Thom for his love, support, inspiration and wonderful wit.

Contents

I'm Having a Baby— Help Me, Lord!

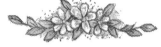

"Congratulations, Cathy. You're going to have a baby," the nurse told me quite calmly.

I stared at her, stunned. I had come for a checkup.

"Are you sure?" I asked. "I don't think it's possible for me to be pregnant."

My doctor, a kind man who delivered our first three children, confirmed the results. "You could probably write a book on pregnancy, so I don't think I need to make a speech about getting plenty of rest, eating right, and so on...."

I left the doctor feeling surprised, shocked, perhaps a bit overwhelmed. Not knowing what to say, I prayed: "God, please help me. I love my children. I know babies are gifts from You. I know my life is in Your hands. But why, Lord? Why this baby now?"

Sunshine streamed through my windshield on that beautiful summer day, warming my body and reaching into my heart. Conflicting emotions churned inside me. Surprise and excitement blended together with a touch of worry and fear.

"What's there to worry about?" I thought. "I love having babies!" A surge of happiness seemingly washed away the anxiety.

Laughing and crying simultaneously, Scripture passages I had read over and over during previous pregnancies flooded my mind:

"Blessed is the man who fears the Lord, who finds great delight in his commands. His children will be mighty in the land; the generation of the upright will be blessed."

This passage, Psalm 112:1-2, was one I read many times while I was pregnant with our third child, Benjamin.

"Children are a gift from God; they are his reward" (Ps. 127:3, TLB) jumped out at me again and again while I carried David, our second baby.

9

"And thy children shall be taught of the Lord, and great shall be the peace of thy children," Isaiah declares to God's chosen people (54:13, KJV). I saw the reality of this verse—which my husband, Thom, and I prayed together during my first pregnancy—in our daughter, Holly Lou. Her sweet spirit brings peace to herself and those around her.

As these and other Scripture verses came to mind, I was reminded of how much fun it is to be pregnant. My husband, normally very nice, is exceptionally sweet and supportive. We pray together often; he encourages me to get plenty of rest and to do my exercises. When I begin to look like a large pumpkin, he tells me I look like a beautiful pumpkin. Sure, I'm uncomfortable at times, but overall my hair shines and my cheeks glow. I eat nutritious things, exercise and declare a moratorium on coffee, diet drinks, donuts and other generally unhealthy items.

Best of all, with each pregnancy I come closer to the Lord. Another life is growing inside me. I need God! He helps me through fear and doubt, and actually directs and teaches me to rely on Him one day at a time. As I draw near to Him, He draws near to me. Isaiah 40:11 says the Lord "shall gently lead those that are with young" (KJV). That's me!

Continuing on the drive home from the doctor, the Lord impressed upon my mind that the child forming within me was created in His image. I thought about that for a while and, knowing that God is love, was comforted that this child conceived in love would surely bring more of God's love into the world.

"I could write a book about having a baby," I announced to no one but the Lord. "But it won't be on how to choose a layette or an obstetrician, or what to eat and what to wear. I want to tell the world how wonderful it is to know You are near me, Lord."

There are dozens and dozens of books available on the medical, emotional and physical aspects of pregnancy. I collected a number of them during previous pregnancies. I've read some books with inspirational poems and thoughts and some that deal with doctrinal issues of women, childbirth and motherhood; but I've seen very few that emphasize spiritual preparation for childbirth and parenting.

We are raising another generation! It is our responsibility to equip our children spiritually, to furnish them with tools to continue building the church. Baby blankets and pacifiers will fade away, but the kingdom of God will last forever. "One generation shall praise thy works to another, and shall declare thy mighty acts," the Bible says in Psalm 145:4 (KJV). One of my jobs as a mother is to tell my children of the goodness of God.

Through Bible reading, prayer, praise and worship, and meditation, parents prepare themselves and begin to lay a spiritual foundation that through their growing families could impact succeeding generations.

I have kept a diary throughout each pregnancy, recording my thoughts, feelings, prayers and answers to prayers, as well as tracking the physical changes in my body. Riding in the car on the way home from the doctor that day, I couldn't wait to read my journal entries for the days on which I discovered I was pregnant with the other children. For each pregnancy, I typed lists of Scripture verses, wisdom followed for ages by Jewish mothers, and taped them to my bathroom wall. Several times a day these verses taught, inspired, reassured and blessed me. The thought occurred to me that, if I was anxious to reread these special verses and journals, perhaps other mothers would benefit from them.

I've enjoyed healthy, happy pregnancies that culminated in fast, easy deliveries. I think the ease I've enjoyed in pregnancy comes from a variety of factors, including a belief in natural childbirth and the physical preparation it involves, an incredibly wonderful, supportive husband, proper diet and exercise, and perhaps a body build that is conducive to childbearing. Who knows?

But when my water breaks and "push comes to shove," I want to know that I'm right with God, that He is with me, blessing me, helping me and my child, whether labor and delivery are easy or hard. The peace of God that passes my human understanding has been ever-present with me through labor and delivery so far. This peace has allowed me to relax, to rest in God's strength, diminishing fear and tension, the main culprits of pain during labor.

"God does not show favoritism," says Peter in Acts 10:34. The promises in the Bible apply to all whose faith is in God. What He has done for me, He will do for others who draw close to Him.

Does this mean every pregnant woman will have nine months of comfort and fun? I doubt it. We're all different; each pregnant woman has unique quirks, cravings and feelings. But I guarantee that God knows and understands our quirks better than anyone. This is a time when we will want to be very close to our Creator.

I don't know if you will be as I've been in the past and have a fast, easy, unmedicated delivery and a beautifully healthy baby. I'm going to be praying for that end in this pregnancy, and I hope and pray the same for you.

Prayer starter: Help me, Lord. I'm going to have a baby. I need You to lead and guide me. I pray You'll bless and protect the child I'm carrying. Please bless and protect all the pregnant mothers and their children. Use me, Lord, as You see fit to encourage, strengthen and equip myself, my family and my sisters in Christ as we raise another generation to praise You.

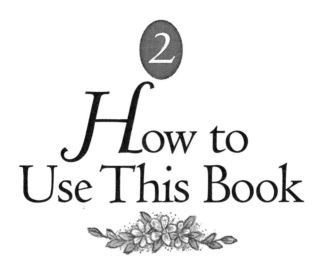

How to Use This Book

If you're reading this book, thank you! You are an answer to prayer. If you are pregnant or want to be, congratulations! I give you a pat on the back. Pregnancy is such an exciting, exhilarating time! It's an important, special time. Both a baby and parents are in the process of development. Whether this is your first or fourteenth baby, God has blessed and entrusted you with the awesome responsibility of nurturing a child created in His image. You are wise to draw close to the Lord at this time and to get serious about spending quality time with Him.

Join me one day at a time as we gain weight, buy maternity clothes, visit the doctor, make arrangements with grandparents, choose a layette, pray, cry, laugh, sing and celebrate the creation of a new life together. I'm pregnant as I write this, and I'm praying for all of you who will ever read these devotions. The daily thoughts and meditations are a culmination of my four pregnancies, the stories and anecdotes of friends, and general thoughts I hope will draw you and your baby close to God.

After the next chapter, there are 266 days of devotions which are loosely arranged according to month. Each chapter contains an overview of the child's development during that month, followed by daily devotions designed for that time period. We're going to pray for your child's heart as it begins to beat, for internal organs, toes, lips, fingers, hands and feet— all the baby's biological development. At the end of each chapter you will find space to record your thoughts, prayers, physical development, answers to prayers, and revelations.

Each day I include a Scripture quotation, a meditation and a prayer starter. I hope you utilize this material to supplement your time with the Lord.

Whatever stage of development your child is in as you begin this book, I urge you to read the first three chapters through the daily devotions to the day you calculate you're currently on. Take some time to jot down your experiences. What was your reaction and your husband's reaction to the news of your pregnancy? What names are you considering? What did you think after your first visit to the doctor? Were any of the Bible verses or the meditations helpful or encouraging to you?

This book assumes a normal pregnancy, free of complications. The 266 devotions represent the average biological timetable for the development of a baby from the day of conception. The American College of Obstetrics and Gynecology estimates that eighty percent of expectant mothers give birth between thirty-eight and forty-two weeks from the first day of their last period. Another ten percent give birth before thirty-eight weeks, and ten percent give birth after forty-two weeks.

Of course there is no such thing as a "normal pregnancy," because every mother and every child are unique. This book is not a medical text, so don't be upset if your baby is born on day 268 or day 292. If you're trying to get pregnant, the day of conception should fall approximately fourteen days after the beginning of your last period. Start reading on day one—the day you believe you conceive your child. If you do not conceive that day, or month, try all over again! There's no rule against peeking ahead.

God knows and loves you. He has blessed you now with new life for His purposes. Regardless of the circumstances surrounding your pregnancy, be of good cheer. First Peter 2:9 says, "You are a chosen people, a royal priesthood, a holy nation, a people belonging to God, that you may declare the praises of him who called you out of darkness into his wonderful light."

Just as a baby lives in darkness for nine months then is born into the light of the world, God's people must be called spiritually out of darkness into light. In the third chapter of John, Jesus calls this spiritual awakening being "born again." "Flesh gives birth to flesh," referring to childbirth, Jesus says, "but the Spirit gives birth to spirit."

If you have been born of the Spirit, the Bible promises that this book contains are for you to cling to, meditate upon, believe and receive. If you are not sure if you're born of the Spirit, open your mind and your heart, then join with us, sisters in the family of God, as we prepare for childbirth. Give God a chance now, when He has blessed you with another life and charged you with the responsibility of motherhood.

I also hope that, if possible, your husband will join with you as you exercise your spiritual muscles and prepare for parenthood. Encourage him to read these devotions with you. Having his support, understanding and encouragement will be a strength to you. Don't forget—he has needs, too!

*B*e Prepared

My motto is **PREPARE**:

Pray for your unborn child daily. Pray for God's guidance in regard to motherhood. Pray for the baby's father, grandparents, older brothers and sisters, aunts, uncles. Pray for the atmosphere into which the child will be born and grow. Pray, pray, pray! "The prayer of a righteous man is powerful and effective," according to James 5:16.

Pray with your mate, and other children if you have them. Jesus says in Matthew 18:19, "I tell you that if two of you on earth agree about anything you ask for, it will be done for you by my Father in heaven." Of course, your family will want to "agree" with you in prayer concerning the newest member of the family. In the following verse Jesus goes on to say, "For where two or three come together in my name, there am I with them." By praying together in Jesus' name, your family invites and involves the very presence of the Lord. The daily meditations in this book contain "prayer starters." I hope you will continue to pray about the needs and concerns that are unique to your circumstances.

When you pray, take time to listen. Be still before the Lord.

Read! As you read and meditate upon the Bible, God will speak to you through it. Read this book and the daily thoughts and meditations. Read books that give advice and information on nutrition, exercise, choosing a doctor, deciding how and where to have your child. I've included a list of references that helped me. Correct information is important. The Bible says, "You will know the truth and the truth will set you free" (John 8:32). The truth is, God made our bodies marvelously to bear children. Understanding the biological process of childbirth set me free from the fear of the unknown and the fear of other people's awful stories.

15

When my last baby was born, I could feel and envision his descent through the birth canal in the midst of my most intense labor. The result? A smooth, easy delivery.

Eat right and exercise. The child within you deserves a healthy start in life. There is plenty of literature for expectant mothers on what to eat. Ask your doctor for information if necessary. Take supplemental vitamins according to your doctor's instructions. Drink plenty of pure water. (Believe me, it helps prevent constipation.) I've exercised throughout each pregnancy according to the instructions for natural deliveries outlined in *Husband-Coached Childbirth* (Harper & Row) by Robert A. Bradley. Remember: labor means work, not necessarily pain.

Take care of yourself. Take care of the child growing inside of you. Treat your body with respect. "Know ye not that ye are the temple of God, and that the Spirit of God dwelleth in you?" (1 Cor. 3:16, KJV).

Praise the Lord continually. Sing—"make melody in your heart," Scripture says. A tape of praise music played in the background on that beautiful summer day I found out I was pregnant. I sang along with praise music as Thom drove me to the hospital while in labor. Now I rock my baby to sleep, singing the praises of God. Praising God invites Him to dwell in our hearts. Praise is a spiritual weapon to fight off evil that cannot remain where God's Spirit is present. The Lord inhabits the praises of His people, the Bible says in Psalm 22:3.

Accept yourself and your unborn child. God loves you just the way you are. What good does worrying do at this point? Give any fears or feelings of inadequacy to God. Did you drink alcohol, sit in a hot tub or take cold medicine before you knew you were pregnant? Worrying will not help you now. God will surround you with peace and love if you allow Him to. I had plenty of things I could have worried about when I was surprised by this pregnancy; you may have also. But remember, God is blessing us with babies to love, nourish, discipline, teach and raise to adulthood. Accept yourself and your current condition. You may as well face it—you've got a job assignment that will last a lifetime. You're another human being's only mom!

Record this special time in your life. At the end of each chapter I've left space for you to fill in your thoughts and ideas. How much weight have you gained? How do you feel? Are you craving particular foods? What are your thoughts and prayers? Have any special Scripture verses come to mind? When did you first feel the baby move? Keep a journal of your pregnancy either briefly in this book or in depth. I guarantee from experience that the Lord will speak to you through His Word during this time. Later your thoughts will be a precious prebirth baby book for your child. The Lord told the prophet Jeremiah, "Before I formed thee in the belly, I knew thee; and before thou camest forth out of the womb I sanctified thee, and I ordained thee a prophet unto the nations" (1:5, KJV). God surely has plans for our babies, even while they're in our wombs.

Encourage your unborn child, yourself, your husband, other children, parents and close friends, with Scripture verses, your prayers and your thoughts during pregnancy. Read out loud to your baby. Sing to him or her. The environment into which your baby is born is so important. Your encouragement to others will set the tone for a peaceful, godly atmosphere for your child. If you have other children, your verbal assurance that they, too, are special and loved will provide additional security, minimizing negative feelings toward the new baby.

*B*e Fruitful and Multiply

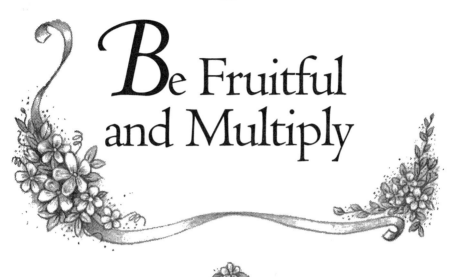

D A Y S   1 – 2 9

MONTH ONE On the day of conception, about fourteen days after your last period, male sperm unites with a female egg. The resulting single cell is, in its embryonic stage, a totally unique individual complete with all its genetic information that determines hair and eye color, size, shape and distinguishing characteristics. Now is not the time to pray for a blue-eyed blonde or a raven-haired boy. Even in one tiny cell the child is what it is.

The fertilized egg travels through the Fallopian tube to the uterus where it attaches itself to the uterine wall and grows rapidly. The heart, brain, lungs and digestive and nervous systems begin to develop. On or around the twenty-fifth day, the heart begins to beat! By the end of the first month, the child measures around one quarter of an inch and weighs seven ten-thousandths of an ounce.

Two weeks or so after conception you will more than likely miss your regular menstrual cycle. Other physical indications of pregnancy during the first three months include frequent urination, swelling and tenderness in the breasts, and possibly nausea and fatigue. A woman's entire body changes throughout pregnancy as her blood supply and hormone levels increase and milk ducts move into action. These physical changes account for much of the tiredness, emotional changes and perhaps food cravings. Add this to the joy and excitement, or perhaps fear and dread or maybe even ambivalence to pregnancy, and you have a woman who needs love, understanding, kindness and tenderness from her husband and family.

Anyone suspecting she's pregnant should stop smoking and drinking alcohol. Consult a physician about any prescribed or over-the-counter medications. Whatever you eat, drink, smoke or inhale you share with the tiny baby inside your womb.

Let's begin our 266-day journey together now, learning about ourselves and the growing child inside of us. As I write, I don't know if my baby is a boy or a girl. I refer to the child interchangeably as "he" or "she."

Prayer starter: Father, in Jesus' name I pray You will bless the fruit of my womb and touch every developing part of this baby.

DAY

1 "Be fruitful and multiply" *(Gen. 1:22; 9:1; 35:11, KJV).*

I've heard it said that this is one command mankind has no trouble obeying. Surely, conceiving a child is a joyful, pleasurable event in a loving marriage. God first told Adam and Eve, then Noah's children and finally Israel to "be fruitful and multiply." The earth is now thoroughly populated, yet there is a greater need than ever for men, women and children to bring God's light and love into a dark and troubled world. God seeks people to love, obey and serve Him willingly.

Prayer starter: Lord, my husband and I are ready to be parents. We are willing to produce children who will be dedicated to You. We ask for Your blessings as we come together in love to produce a child. Help us. Give us wisdom and strength. We love and trust You, Lord, and believe You will bless us with children in Your perfect timing.

DAY
2

"But the fruit of the Spirit is love, joy, peace, patience, kindness, goodness, faithfulness, gentleness and self-control"
(Gal. 5:22).

As women preparing to become mothers, we're obeying God's
command to be fruitful—to bear children. As we plan biological
children, we should also pray about producing spiritual fruit in our
own lives. For the next nine months, we have the opportunity to concentrate on developing the nine fruits of the Spirit in our character,
praying that these fruits will also be manifested in our babies' lives.

This month let's work on love. It is hoped that your baby conceived in love will grow in love. The root of the Hebrew word for
"womb" means "to love." Our wombs are places of love.

The Bible says that God is love. Day by day, if we are conformed
into the image of Christ, we become more loving. Christ said there
is no greater love than to lay down one's life for friends.

In 1 Corinthians 13:4-8 (NAS), the apostle Paul describes the
attributes of love: "Love is patient, love is kind, and is not jealous;
love does not brag and is not arrogant, does not act unbecomingly;
it does not seek its own, is not provoked, does not take into account
a wrong suffered, does not rejoice in unrighteousness, but rejoices
with the truth; bears all things, believes all things, hopes all things,
endures all things. Love never fails."

By rereading this passage, putting your own name where you see
the word "love," you may get a revelation of how God wants you
to love and where your life needs a little work. I struggle with the
need for approval and acceptance from others. When I'm pregnant
especially, I get my feelings hurt. I need to work on this reaction
because "love doesn't take into account a wrong suffered."

*Prayer starter: Father, help me this month to learn how to love as
You love. Cultivate the fruit of love in my life. Teach me to love the
way I should. Forgive me when I act unloving. Instill Your love into
my children.*

DAY
3
"My beloved is mine, and I am his" *(Song 2:16, KJV).*

What fun it has been, getting to know this man, this husband of mine. After years of searching, I know I married the man of my dreams: kind and loving, sensitive and strong. I'm thankful to God for this friend and lover who understands and encourages me. I try to help him, as he helps me, to be all God wants us to be. It is an exciting adventure to enjoy parenthood together.

Prayer starter: Lord, our marriage is dedicated to You. Help us to be the parents You want us to be. Teach us, prepare us, show us how to be a good father and mother. We thank You for each other.

DAY
4
"If you abide in Me, and My words abide in you, ask whatever you wish, and it shall be done for you" *(John 15:7, NAS).*

How can I abide in God and have His words abide in me? I must keep God first in my life. I need to communicate with Him continually to build a strong, loving, personal relationship with Him. My husband and I have each other to remind and reassure one another of God's loving presence and direction in our lives. We attend a closely knit local church where we have fellowship with other Christians. Yet I need to have God's Word abiding in *me.* I need to abide in God *as an individual* if I am to be one with Him.

Prayer starter: Father, help me to be diligent in my Bible reading and prayer. I treasure the time we have together, yet so often the cares of the world carry me away from You. You know that I desire to have a baby. Most of all I want to walk in the path You have set for me. I put all my hopes and desires into Your hands.

DAY
5   "Parents are the pride of their children" *(Prov. 17:6).*

My five-year-old's teacher told me that Holly often brags about her parents: "My daddy is so funny....My mommy tells such good stories....My daddy is so strong he can lift me up by my feet!" I guess it's pretty common for children to have pride in their parents. I hope I'll have a good relationship with my children all of our lives. I want my kids to be proud of me, just as I know that I'll be proud of them.

Prayer starter: Lord, I want my children to be proud of me. Mold me into the kind of mother You want me to be. Bless my husband and help him grow into a loving father. Give us favor in the eyes of our children and in Your eyes, Lord.

DAY
6   "For God hath not given us the spirit of fear; but of power, and of love, and of a sound mind" *(2 Tim. 1:7, KJV).*

I confess: I am afraid. I'm afraid of the responsibility of being a parent. I'm afraid of childbirth. I'm afraid a baby may change my life in ways with which I'm not prepared to cope. I'm afraid of failure, of my inability to perform all the expectations I have of myself and that others have of me. Yet I know that my fears are not from the Lord. They're *my* fears, and as I die daily to myself I can receive from God the attributes He gives me to do His will: power, love and a sound mind.

Prayer starter: Lord, please help me know that You are with me and that You understand my fears. Once again I lay my fears before You and pray that You will remove them, replacing them with Your power, love and wisdom.

DAY
7

"Blessed is he whose help is the God of Jacob, whose hope is in the Lord his God, the Maker of heaven and earth, the sea, and everything in them—the Lord who remains faithful forever" *(Ps. 146:5-6).*

Sometime around the fourth day, the cluster of cells that forms your child travels through the Fallopian tube to the uterus. After several more days, the baby becomes attached to the uterine lining where it remains, growing rapidly until its birth.

Our God who crafted the universe also marvelously designed our bodies to reproduce. The uterus is quite prepared to nurture the baby. As the cluster of cells which is already distinguished as your unique child burrows into the uterine lining, tiny blood vessels are broken. These provide nutrients for the baby and perhaps a little spotting for the mother.

In each of my pregnancies, I was either amazed or alarmed at the sign of this tiny bit of blood. This time I recorded the spotting in my diary, not guessing I was pregnant but wanting to have accurate information to tell my doctor if necessary.

I trust in God; He created my body, soul and spirit. The Bible says we who trust in Him are blessed. I trust right now, even when I'm not sure what's happening, that He is positioning my baby carefully in the precise spot for healthy development over the next nine months.

Prayer starter: Lord, my trust is in You who made the heavens and the earth, the sea and everything in them. I pray that You will guide this baby to the exact spot in the uterine wall that is best for his growth and development in the womb. I pray You'll bless and protect this baby now and forever.

DAY
8

"At the name of Jesus every knee should bow, in heaven and on earth and under the earth, and every tongue confess that Jesus Christ is Lord, to the glory of God the Father" *(Phil. 2:10).*

24

Through the work in radio and newspaper that my husband and I do in Pittsburgh, we have sponsored many Christian concerts and rallies over the years. I'm always interested to meet the various musicians, evangelists and artists with whom we work behind the scenes "with their hair down."

I don't like to judge, trying to remember that I have little idea of what it must be like living on the road, pouring myself out daily before auditoriums full of people. It does seem, however, that some are in the ministry to glorify themselves, not the Lord. Others are willing to come into a city, sleep on church floors and eat what is provided, trusting God to take care of them.

One group we've worked with a half dozen times or so is the 2nd Chapter of Acts. On stage or off, the members of this group lift up the Lord, not themselves and the remarkable talent they possess. I was touched at one of their concerts in the late 1970s. During a time of worship and praise, sisters Annie Herring and Nellie Griesen dropped to their knees before the Lord. I had never seen anyone do this on stage. As I watched, I realized the women were not thinking, Oh my, what's this going to look like to the crowd? They were totally caught up in leading worship in His awesome presence in the auditorium.

There will come a day when every knee will bow and every tongue confess that Jesus Christ is Lord. Throughout eternity He will reign. Those who believe that Jesus is the Savior, the Messiah, need to have eternal eyes and walk in the ways of God's kingdom. I want to be able to say openly to my children, "Come, let us bow down in worship, let us kneel before the Lord our Maker" (Ps. 95:6).

Prayer starter: Father, we humbly bow before You, acknowledging You as our Creator and the One who is forming the child within. We love You, worship You, praise and adore You. I pray for the baby I'm carrying that she, too, will have a heart to worship and praise You, Lord.

DAY
9

"Anyone who loves his father or mother more than me is not worthy of me; anyone who loves his son or daughter more than me is not worthy of me; and anyone who does not take

his cross and follow me is not worthy of me" *(Matt. 10:37-38).*

The woman in front of me in line at the bank is holding a beautiful baby girl. Her big blue eyes, peeking out from a pink ruffled bonnet, dance with delight at the sights and sounds around her. What a treasure! How easy it is to fall in love with a baby! When our little Holly was about the same age as this child, I remember thinking that perhaps I loved her more than anything on the face of the earth. For six or seven months my life revolved around her eating, sleeping, playing. The same thing happened when the two boys were infants and dependent upon me.

The kind of love I have for my children is different from any love I've ever known in my life. I'm protective of them and shudder to think any harm would come to them. I wonder how a new baby will affect my relationship with God, my husband and our other children?

Prayer starter: Help me, Father, to use godly wisdom in all of my relationships, whether they're with children, husband, relatives or friends. I want You to be first in my life always.

DAY 10

"I will instruct you and teach you in the way which you should go. I will counsel you with My eye upon you" *(Ps. 32:8, NAS).*

My sister, who is expecting, avoids caffeine and fatty foods. Her boss recently brought out-of-the-oven donuts and pastries and fresh brewed coffee to work to share with the staff. Her mouth watering, my sister bravely turned down the tempting treats. Just as "no, thank you" rolled off her lips, the baby kicked her in the ribs. She interpreted this as a sign that she should indulge in a donut dunked in coffee. So she did.

I believe strongly that women should monitor what they eat and drink during pregnancy. But there is a point where a little moderation with no-no foods could be tolerated by the baby and enjoyed by mom. A donut has about three hundred calories of non-nutritious white flour, white sugar, shortening and grease. Too many donuts will simply add weight that will be difficult to lose after having a child. Think about that before you say yes to an ooey-gooey donut or fall for the myth that all pregnant women crave sweets at 3:00 a.m

Prayer starter: Lord, I commit my eating and drinking habits to You. I trust in Your counsel and I'm thankful that You are watching me.

DAY 11

"He will love you and bless you and increase your numbers. He will bless the fruit of your womb" *(Deut. 7:13).* **"The fruit of your womb will be blessed"** *(Deut. 28:4).*

God gives promises of blessings to His people. These blessings have a condition, however. The promises of God apply to those who choose to obey Him. "If you fully obey the Lord your God and carefully follow all his commands I give you today, the Lord your God will set you high above all the nations of the earth. All these blessings will come upon you and accompany you if you obey the Lord your God" (Deut. 28:1-2).

Prayer starter: Lord, empower me by Your Spirit to say yes to Your will and no to evil and my own selfish desires. I want to walk in a covenant of love and obedience to You.

DAY 12

"Be perfect, therefore, as your heavenly Father is perfect" *(Matt. 5:48).*

I have struggled in several areas of my life to be perfect in my own strength. I desire to be the perfect wife, the perfect mother, the perfect writer. I cannot be perfect. Over and over again I make mistakes.

There was one man who lived a perfect life. He obeyed all of God's laws and never made a mistake. This man, Jesus, was also God's Son. Jesus chose to pay the penalty for my imperfection by dying on the cross. God accepted this sacrifice for the imperfections of all mankind and raised Jesus from the dead. By doing so, the perfection of Jesus Christ, His righteousness, became available for the entire human race. By receiving Jesus Christ into my life, I accept His righteousness. I can be perfect, my imperfections forgiven in God's eyes, because Jesus Christ paid the price for me. Luke quotes the words of the resurrected Christ: "Yes, it was written long ago that the Messiah must suffer and die and rise again from the dead on the third day; and that this message of salvation should be taken from Jerusalem to all the nations: There is forgiveness of sins for all who turn to me" (Luke 24:46-47, TLB).

Prayer starter: Father, I thank You for Jesus, for what He did for me. I confess my frustrations in struggling for perfection and righteousness in my own strength. Fill me, Lord, anew with Your Spirit this day, so that I can walk in Your way and be perfect in Your eyes.

DAY 13

"And all things you ask in prayer, believing, you shall receive" *(Matt. 21:22, NAS).*

Every night we tuck our three little ones in bed with stories, prayers and tapes of soft music to fall asleep to. Last night Holly prayed last: "Lord, please let me have a baby sister and a house big enough to fit the refrigerator into the kitchen." Thom and I bit our lips to keep from giggling. Holly's been praying for a baby sister for a long time. She adores her two little brothers and never once said she wished they were girls instead of boys. But the part about the refrigerator is new. When the prayers were over and the hugs and kisses distributed to all, Thom said gently to Holly, "God knows what's best for our family. Do you know that?"

"Yes, Daddy."

"So we'll just trust Him about everything in our lives: houses, babies, where we work and where we play. OK?"

"OK," Holly replied sleepily. "I did want God to know that I want a baby sister...and it would be nice if our refrigerator would fit in the kitchen...," she murmured softly before sleep shut her beautiful brown eyes.

Prayer starter: Lord, we acknowledge You as the Creator of all life. We trust You to bless us with children in Your timing. We commit to love, nourish, discipline and train the child You give us, regardless of his or her gender and characteristics.

DAY 14

"Finally, brothers, whatever is true, whatever is noble, whatever is right, whatever is admirable...if anything is excellent or praiseworthy—think about such things" *(Phil. 4:8).*

I was born, the fourth of five children, in Pittsburgh's large women's hospital. With my father by her side, my mother delivered me under the covers in her bed without a doctor. A young resident had examined Mom and predicted my arrival was hours away. But a few minutes after the doctor left, to the surprise of everyone except my mother and me, I gently popped out. Mother didn't make it to the delivery room until after my birth.

I've heard that story told with pride all of my life. I'm thankful my parents considered childbirth to be a joyful event, not a torture session. I'm also grateful that they remind me often that I was wanted and very much loved. I found out later that not all of my mother's deliveries were quite so fast and simple, yet she never has been one to dwell on the negative. She looks on the sunny side of life and has helped me to do the same.

Prayer starter: Lord, help me to think thoughts that are lovely, true and right. Guide me by Your Spirit away from thoughts that would tear down my faith and confidence in You.

DAY 15

"Train a child in the way he should go, and when he is old he will not turn from it" *(Prov. 22:6).*

Right past the cereal section of the supermarket, a small child wails. Throwing himself to the floor with drama, he screams hysterically, "I want Captain Crunch! I want Captain Crunch!"

"No! I said no!" the young mother replies with frustration. The child continues his tantrum. "If you don't get up right now, I'm going to beat your bottom!" the mother warns. The little boy cries on, undaunted by his mother's threats. Then, sure enough, she pulls down his pants and spanks him firmly, right in front of the Cheerios.

To spank or not to spank, that is the question. With all the news of child abuse, I hate to hear about anyone's spanking a child. Yet, clearly, children must be disciplined. "Speak softly and carry a big stick," Theodore Roosevelt's oft-quoted foreign-policy motto, has been a key to our family's discipline. A gentle yet firm and consistent parent commands respect, especially if he or she carries a big stick. I try to keep a wooden spoon with me, not so much as a means of punishment but as a reminder of who the boss is.

Thom and I did not adopt our disciplinary policy by chance or accident. We read a variety of books and came together as husband and wife to decide how we felt we best could "train our children in the way they should go." Particularly helpful have been James Dobson's books, especially *Dare to Discipline* (Tyndale House), and his magazines, radio broadcasts and videotapes. I rely on Dr. Grace Ketterman's books, in particular, *The Complete Book of Baby and Child Care* (Revell). And I have learned many insights from a women's Bible study which our pastor's wife taught, using the book *A Woman's Workshop on Mastering Motherhood* (Zondervan) by Barbara Bush.

Prayer starter: Lord, I pray for all the mothers and fathers who are trying to raise their children right now. Help us to train these little ones in the way You want them to go. Give us wisdom to discipline our children and to raise them in godliness.

DAY 16

"Like arrows in the hand of a warrior, so are the children of one's youth. How blessed is the man whose quiver is full of them" *(Ps. 127:4-5, NAS).*

Our third child, Benjamin, was conceived on Valentine's Day. I knew I was pregnant. I felt pregnant from the first day. I waited about two weeks after the date of conception, then bought a home pregnancy test. It was negative. The next day I bought another one. (They're available at most drugstores and very affordable.) The test was negative again and my husband kidded me. "You're not pregnant! You're imagining it." The next day I had a blood test. It was positive! I ended up spending a total of thirty dollars. The satisfaction of detecting my pregnancy as early as possible was well worth the money. I want to be well-prepared and healthy before bringing a baby into the world.

Prayer starter: Lord, help me during these childbearing years to care for my health especially well, so that I can in turn produce strong, healthy children.

DAY
17
"She girdeth her loins with strength, and strengtheneth her arms" *(Prov. 31:17, KJV).*

According to the dictionary, the loin is the "lower part of the back on either side of the backbone between the hipbones and the ribs." By her ninth month a pregnant woman better have strong loins or she'll have a tough time getting out of bed, let alone walking around all day with twenty to thirty pounds of extra weight on her. Now is the time to start strengthening those loins! And every mother needs to have strong arms. Perhaps for two years we carry our babies while performing many routine tasks. You can get the idea of how strong your arms will need to be by carrying a ten-pound sack of potatoes around with you while you work.

I like the Amplified Bible's translation of this verse: "She girds herself with strength [spiritual, mental and physical fitness for her God-given task] and makes her arms strong and firm." Our bodies need to be strong for the God-given task of motherhood. We'll be better equipped to have and care for our children if our bodies are healthy.

Prayer starter: Lord, with my days so filled with activity, please help me carve out some time to exercise. Help me also to have the diligence and discipline to strengthen my physical body.

DAY 18

"Husbands ought to love their wives as their own bodies. He who loves his wife loves himself" *(Eph. 5:28).*

I went to the doctor because I felt a little strange. I had not had a checkup since the last baby had been born, and I wanted to make sure everything was OK. Neither Thom nor I remotely suspected that I could be pregnant. But I am. After my ride home, talking to the Lord and trying to figure out why I was going to have another baby, I went straight to the office to tell Thom the news.

I thought about the first time I found out I was pregnant: Thom picked me up and twirled me around the lobby of the radio station where we worked and lived. We took a photograph of the positive home pregnancy test and rejoiced together. Then we excitedly shared the news with our good friend and office manager, Barb, who joined us in celebrating and praising God.

I did not envision the same reception this time. Thom and I had been offered jobs in another state and we were contemplating a move. Our living quarters, already bursting at the seams with a family of five, were not large enough to hold one more baby. Our refrigerator didn't fit in the kitchen, which for some reason had become a prayer concern for Holly. Thom bore a lot of pressure producing the regional Christian newspaper we publish; we distribute the newspaper free as a non-profit ministry, and we struggle to make ends meet. I was afraid that the news of my pregnancy would make him unhappy.

When I arrived at the office, I called him into the hallway so we could be alone. I grabbed him around the neck and whispered in his ear, "We're going to have a baby." He did not hesitate even a moment. He picked me up, twirled me around the hall and said, "Oh good! I love babies!"

I cried. Then we prayed together, dedicating our new baby to God and turning over our unspoken worries to Him. Then we told the happy news to Barb, who is still our close friend and office manager. I know that she, too, wondered how in the world we would make it financially, physically, emotionally—having our fourth baby in six years. Yet she praised God and congratulated us.

Prayer starter: Father, thank You for a loving, sensitive husband. Thank You for the love and encouragement of friends. Bless this child growing rapidly inside of me and help me to cast all my cares on You.

DAY 19

"Who may ascend the hill of the Lord? Who may stand in his holy place? He who has clean hands and a pure heart..." *(Ps. 24:3).*

My little ones learned a song in Sunday school, sung to the tune of "If You're Happy and You Know It, Clap Your Hands." It goes like this: "Oh, be careful, little hands, what you do. Oh, be careful, little hands, what you do, for the Father up above is looking down on you in love. Oh, be careful, little hands, what you do." The song goes through various body parts reminding eyes to be careful what they see, ears to be careful what they hear, and mouth to be careful what it says. When we've got Jesus living inside our hearts, His Spirit will guide us, so that all we do brings honor to Him.

Prayer starter: Father, I pray that You will help me by Your Spirit to guard my thoughts, words and actions so that my heart remains pure and my hands clean. I pray for the child growing inside of me that even as the little hands are forming and the heart develops You will bless them and protect them from evil.

DAY 20

"Then he opened their minds so they could understand the Scriptures" *(Luke 24:45).*

The disciples were frightened when Jesus appeared to them after the resurrection. Was this a ghost, or were their minds playing games? Jesus explained that His resurrection had been foretold through the prophets. Then He opened their minds so that the disciples could understand what had occurred.

As a woman expecting a child, I sometimes have frightening thoughts, even though I know the Lord is with me and that He's told me to "fear not." I pray that during this pregnancy God will open my mind just as He opened the minds of the disciples, so that I'll understand the meaning of His Word and have the power by His Spirit to apply it to my life and to the life of my baby.

Prayer starter: Father, open my mind to the truth of Your Word. Bless me with discernment and wisdom as I read and meditate on the Scriptures. Help me in the coming months to learn from You and trust that You've got my life and the life of my child in Your hands. Lord, I pray that this baby from the earliest moment possible will have a mind open to the Scriptures.

DAY 21

"Call to me and I will answer you and tell you great and unsearchable things you do not know" *(Jer. 33:3).*

Prayer is a two-way street. God beckons us to communicate with Him. He also says He will answer us. So often my prayers end up sounding like a gripe session or a grocery list. I need the comfort of going to my loving Father with my needs, hurts and concerns. But I also need to listen; there are so many great and unsearchable things I would like to know.

Today I drove Holly to kindergarten after a hectic morning of bathing, clothing and feeding the family. Holly and I prayed together lifting up the needs of the family and the frustrations of the day. After saying good-bye, I returned to the silent car and felt the presence of the Lord. It was as if He was trying to remind me to "be still and know that I am God." He wanted me to listen.

Prayer starter: Father, forgive me for my self-centeredness that even slips into my prayer life. Teach me to pray so that our communication is indeed a two-way street. As I prepare to have a baby, I want to hear from You.

DAY 22

"But our families will continue; generation after generation will be preserved by your protection" *(Ps. 102:28, TLB).*

Can you envision your family tree with your parents, grandparents and great-grandparents on one side and your husband's parents, grandparents and great-grandparents on the other side? Now put your own face on the tree and picture the generations that will come after you. Some little twig at the end of the family tree, three or four generations from now, could very well spend eternity praising God because you prayed diligently.

I'm excited to know that Christians in my family must have prayed for me sometime. Thom's grandmother told me she prayed for him to find a God-fearing wife even when he was a little boy. I'm an answer to a grandmother's prayer. I owe it to my descendants to pray, pray, pray!

Prayer starter: Lord, I pray not only for the baby growing within me now, but I pray for all my descendants that they'll love and serve You. Teach me to raise my baby with a hunger and thirst for righteousness that will not end with her generation.

DAY 23

"I will try to walk a blameless path, but how I need your help, especially in my own home, where I long to act as I should" *(Ps. 101:2, TLB).*

I'm thankful for my home, but I confess I don't really enjoy spending much time here alone. So often Thom goes out, accomplishing the work he's got to do, meeting interesting people, getting taken to executive lunches in expensive restaurants. I shouldn't complain, because I maintain an active fun schedule with the children inside and outside of the house. But there are days that seem to drag on endlessly. When the mountain of laundry is conquered, it's on to a stack of dirty dishes.

One of my friends, a mother of four, is very excited that a twenty-four-hour grocery store opened near her home. Late at night, with her husband and children fast asleep, she does her grocery shopping all alone. "The sad thing, Cathy, is that it's fun—just to see other adult faces, compare prices, talk to the cashier! Ten years ago, who would have guessed that I would get such a kick out of food shopping?"

With a new baby, I'll be even more confined to my house. I want my time at home with my new baby to be fun, fulfilling and produc-tive. Help me, Lord!

Prayer starter: Father, I will try to walk a blameless path, but how I need Your help, especially in my own home where I long to act as I should. Help me prepare for the days ahead when I'll surely be spending more time here. I know I won't be alone, for You'll be with me.

DAY 24

"Do not be afraid, Mary, you have found favor with God. You will be with child and give birth to a son, and you are to give him the name of Jesus" *(Luke 1:30).*

You may be experiencing an unplanned pregnancy that has you worried, dismayed, disappointed. Perhaps you cannot relate to the jubilation of other pregnant women. Maybe you're alone and afraid that you won't be able to care for your child. Maybe you're a happily married, well-adjusted person who feels a bit overwhelmed with this pregnancy. I think I can understand and relate to how you feel. It's not a bit unusual to have certain misgivings when you're expecting. I believe these feelings should be admitted and expressed to your husband, or to a close friend if you're alone, and especially to the Lord in prayer.

Let me tell you about a young, unwed Jewish girl named Mary. Can you imagine her shock, as a virgin, at hearing the news delivered by an angel that she was pregnant? Mary, who had every reason to be distraught, answered the angel saying, "Be it unto me according to thy word" (Luke 1:38, KJV). She ended up getting a great husband and a baby whom she raised to be the Savior, the Messiah, for all of mankind. She trusted in God's Word and, by doing so, became the example for all of us women. With God, we can do anything if we cast our cares on Him and trust in His Word.

Prayer starter: Father, help me accept Your perfect will for my life. I confess my need for You. I place my life and the life of my baby into Your hands.

DAY
25
"And Jesus increased in wisdom and stature, and in favour with God and man" *(Luke 2:52, KJV).*

"Mom, do you know what I want to be when I grow up?" three-year-old David asked. "I want to be a fireman, a juggler, a lion tamer, a rock star and a wrestling team."

"That's wonderful, honey. Are you going to start training for those jobs now?"

David didn't wait to reply. He picked up a bow and shot make-believe arrows at an invisible monster.

I wonder what little Jesus was like at age three. We don't know much about Him except that He grew wise and strong and was loved by His friends and His heavenly Father. I hope and pray even in the womb that the baby I'm carrying will grow each day in the image of Jesus Christ.

Prayer starter: Lord, bless this baby as he grows, to become more and more like Jesus every day. I pray this child will be wise and strong and that he will be a lovable person.

DAY
26
"Moreover, we have all had human fathers who disciplined us and we respected them for it" *(Heb. 12:9).*

My father never spanked me. He didn't need to. Bearing a resemblance to Superman, my dad's very appearance in a room of noisy, messy, rowdy children commanded enough respect for horseplay to cease. He didn't need to say too much. I remember coming home from a date a few minutes past the 11:00 p.m. curfew time. As my date and I pulled up in front of my house, much to my dismay and fear, Superman was at the window. With stern courtesy, not anger or rage, he confronted me after my date was gone.

"When I say to be home at 11:00, I don't mean 11:15; I don't mean 11:10—I don't mean one minute past 11:00. I want you to be in the house by 11:00. Is that understood?"

I guess so. I was not punished. All the discipline I needed was for this strong, loving father to wait up for me, enforcing the rules we both had agreed upon. I'm quite sure I never came home late again.

Prayer starter: Thank You, Lord, for loving discipline that guides me in the direction You want me to go. Bless my husband with Your wisdom as he grows in his role as a father. I pray this baby will have a teachable spirit.

DAY 27

"How beautiful on the mountains are the feet of those who bring good news" *(Is. 52:7).*

I just love having good news to share! (And my phone bill reflects it.) I have called my parents, three sisters, my brother, my cousin and a few old friends, who live out of town, with the happy news of my pregnancy. Thom has called his sister, grandmother, parents, brother and a cousin or two. New life is good news!

The prophet Isaiah refers to the bearers of good news as the ones who "proclaim peace, who bring good tidings, who proclaim salvation, who say to Zion, 'Your God reigns!' " The announcement of a new child forming is a wonderful opportunity to share with the world the wonder of God's creative power.

Prayer starter: Lord, as I share the news of this baby with my family and friends, fill me with Your joy. Let my friends see Your hand on my life. Bless this baby with beautiful feet that will bring the good news of Your salvation to her generation.

DAY 28

"Thy word is a lamp unto my feet, and a light unto my path" *(Ps. 119:105, KJV).*

Have you ever gone camping and needed to walk along a woodsy path when it was pitch dark? Even walking short distances, it's easy to stray from the path or stumble on a rock. It's just about impossible to see obstacles without a flashlight.

The world is full of darkness, but it's not the kind of darkness that eyes can see; it's spiritual darkness that must be discerned. We have a weapon to combat this darkness, the Word of God. When we read, believe and obey God's Word, He lights our path and keeps us from stumbling and straying from the road we're to travel.

Prayer starter: Lord, help me to be diligent to read Your Word. Even now prepare my baby's heart to love Your Word. Mold her little feet to walk in Your ways.

DAY 29

"For where your treasure is, there your heart will be also" *(Luke 12:34).*

I read an interview with a famous rock star whose music, talents and creativity I admire. This person made a very sad comment, however. He said the only time he felt happy was when he was on stage performing for adoring fans. He lives for his music. What a tragic commentary on his life! For years he put his treasure in "making it" in music. Now that he's made it, his heart can find satisfaction in nothing else.

How many of us treasure our homes, careers or pursuit of riches more than our eternal lives? We are to pursue the kingdom of God first, "circumcising our hearts," Jeremiah says, setting our lives apart from the world in service to God.

Prayer starter: O Father, as my child's little heart begins to beat, please put Your hand of blessing upon him, so that he will store treasures in heaven where neither moth nor rust can destroy. Help me to be a godly example of a mom whose heart seeks first Your kingdom.

What are some of your thoughts? When did you find out you were pregnant? What was your reaction? Your husband's reaction? Have you told the world yet? How much do you weigh? Do you have any food cravings? Do you have special Scripture verses, thoughts or prayers for your unborn child? What specific prayer requests do you have for yourself and your husband as you prepare for parenthood? What special needs do you have for your baby? Have you asked the

Lord to teach you more about the fruit of love? What has He shown you?

Knit Together By God

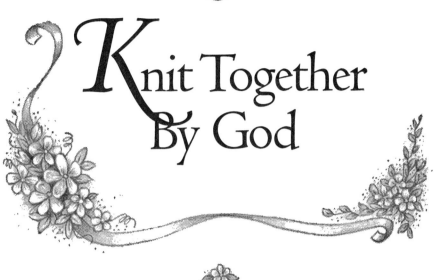

DAYS 30 – 59

MONTH TWO During the second month the baby will grow to about one inch and weigh approximately one third of an ounce. The intestines, internal organs and spinal column form. The brain divides into three parts. Hands, fingers, knees, ankles and toes start to take shape. The long bones begin to develop. The human face appears; ears and hair form.

More than likely, you will schedule your first visit with the doctor this month. Don't expect a big weight gain, but if you're like me, your waist will begin to expand. There's little need for maternity clothes at this stage, but it's nice to feel comfortable. Shirts and blouses worn over apparel with elastic waistlines are all I've ever needed in the early days of pregnancy. Here's a trick for temporarily increasing the waistline of skirts, jeans and slacks that button at the waist. Push one end of a rubber band through the buttonhole, then loop both ends over the button. You've got an expandable waistline with no sewing! Jogging outfits, tunics and oversized shirts are good investments at this point. You'll be able to wear them well into your pregnancy and several months after the baby is born.

Prayer starter: Lord, I pray that Your hand will knit together perfectly every cell of this baby's body.

DAY 30 "You knit me together in my mother's womb" *(Ps. 139:13).*

I learned to knit at my grandmother's knee. I don't practice this craft often. In the past ten years I knit one scarf for my husband. I know just enough to respect those nimble-fingered artists who can create gorgeous sweaters, hats and booties with two needles and some yarn. I watch with awe and wonder as my mother lovingly labors over mittens for her grandchildren.

God's hand is upon us now, knitting together a child with more love and skill than any mother could ever imagine. He marvelously forms each individual. Our bodies are not simple like a sweater made of yarn. Our organs, blood and nervous systems, bones and limbs, skin, hair, teeth—all our parts are complex, brilliantly designed, knit together to function as a unit.

Prayer starter: Lord, I recognize You as the Creator of life. Thank You, Father, that this baby inside me is forming as the result of Your engineering, not by chance or accident. I pray this child will be knit together perfectly, according to Your perfect design, so that he will have health and strength to serve You and Your purposes, Lord.

DAY 31 "The fruit of the Spirit is...joy" *(Gal. 5:22).*

How did you feel when you first suspected you might be pregnant? (Have you begun to feel that yet?) I can go through a list of pregnancies now and remember my various reactions. While my circumstances and feelings differed each time, God always filled me with His supernatural joy.

To know if you have the joy of the Lord in your life, as opposed to the fleeting human feeling of happiness, let's look at some of the opposites of the fruit of joy.

Do you battle the four big D's: discouragement, despair, disillusionment and depression? If you do, you need to work on cultivating the fruit of joy. God is the source of joy, so pray as David did in Psalm 51:12, "Restore unto me the joy of thy salvation" (KJV). Joy from God has nothing to do with circumstances. Look at Paul and Silas in prison in Acts 16. After having been beaten and locked up in jail for preaching, they were filled with joy and sang praises to the Lord! God does not change. His mercy endures forever. When we remember the sacrifice of Christ and that our sins are forever forgiven, we can have joy that brings contentment, happiness, gladness and, yes, *joy* into our lives!

Prayer starter: Lord, help me to look to You and Your salvation for the source of my joy. Forgive me when I grumble and complain, allowing the devil to steal my joy. Give me a rejoicing heart that blesses You and the people around me. Bless my baby with a joyful heart to praise You in all circumstances.

DAY 32

"The eyes of the Lord are in every place, beholding the evil and the good" *(Prov. 15:3, KJV).*

From my kitchen sink I can see out the window into the backyard where the children play. Today I witnessed an unprovoked attack by my son David on the little girl next door. David pushed her down and she cried. He then looked around to see if anyone was watching.

I'm feeling a little woozy these days, and I don't have a reserve of the kind of energy it takes to discipline my active three-year-old. "Lord, help me!" I cried, putting down the final cereal bowl and drying my hands.

"David! Come here right now!" I yelled after seeing that Jessie was not hurt.

David's head drooped as he walked toward me.

"Why is Jessie crying? Did you hurt her?"

"No, Mommy."

"I want you to tell the truth. When you lie, it makes me very angry and it makes the Lord sad. Did you hurt Jessie?"

"I didn't think she would fall down," David whined softly, avoiding eye contact.

"What do you think you could do to make her feel a little better? Could you tell her you're sorry, give her a hug, and tell her you're glad she's your friend?"

"Yes, Mommy."

"That's good. The Lord is happy when you obey your mother and when you are kind to your friends. He'll probably smile when He sees you give Jessie a hug."

David ran back into the yard, told Jessie he was sorry, gave her a hug, then looked around to see if anyone was watching.

Prayer starter: Lord, guide me and all of my children by Your Spirit so that our actions will be pleasing to You, even when no one else is watching. Help me as a mother to teach godly principles to my children, so that they'll grow in Your nurture and admonition. I pray for the baby that I'm carrying, that he will grow to trust and obey You.

DAY 33

"Be joyful always; pray continually; give thanks in all circumstances, for this is God's will for you in Christ Jesus" *(1 Thess. 5:16-18).*

I'm so tired, and my head is pounding. I've got to strip the sheets from Benjamin's crib before the house smells like the bus station floor. How can I be joyful?

Pray continually. "Lord, help me to get the housework done without getting sick."

Give thanks in all circumstances. "Father, thank You for the child You're forming inside of me. My tiredness reminds me that my own body is rearranging to accommodate the needs of this baby. Thank You, Lord, for wonderfully creating me to bear children."

Be joyful. This is difficult. I remember hearing author/evangelist Rebecca Pippert recently. She described a scene in which she asked an African brother casually, "How are you?" The man replied, "Repenting and rejoicing; repenting and rejoicing."

His answer sticks in my mind, especially when I'm feeling a little yucky as I am today. I don't want to be a syrupy Christian who feigns a happy "Praise the Lord" right after I've taken my head out of the toilet. But I want to obey the Scriptures, being joyful and giving thanks continually despite how I feel.

The key to accomplishing this is in those two words the African spoke: "repent" and "rejoice." I realize that I miss the mark, mess up, fall down. I need a Savior. As I repent, I can also rejoice because Christ was crucified with my shortcomings on His back. He rose from the dead, freeing me from all my sins.

Prayer starter: Father, as I go about my day, please help me maintain a joyful attitude knowing that I can rejoice because of what Jesus did for me. I see my sins buried with Christ, and I praise and thank You that since He arose, I can have a pure, righteous, everlasting relationship with You.

DAY 34

"He settles the barren woman in her home as a happy mother of children. Praise the Lord" *(Ps. 113:9).*

My first pregnancy ended at twelve weeks with a miscarriage. The experience was physically excruciating and emotionally draining. Throughout the ordeal, I felt God was very close. My desire to be a mother intensified after the miscarriage. Motherhood and a happy home were not to be taken for granted; these were goals that require work and preparation. I painfully learned that I could not understand the reconciling of the passages "none will miscarry or be barren in your land..." (Ex. 23:26) and "nevertheless not my will, but thine, be done" (Luke 22:42). Thom and I prayed that the Lord would bless us with children and a happy home. These prayers have been answered affirmatively. When I see the Lord face to face, I'll ask Him to explain why I lost our first little one. Until then I must seek to know and do His will.

Prayer starter: Father, I trust You and place my life and the lives of my children anew into Your hands. Thank You for blessing the fruit of my womb and settling me in a happy home.

DAY

35

"Humble yourselves therefore under the mighty hand of God, that he may exalt you in due time" *(1 Pet. 5:6, KJV).*

Just outside of Pittsburgh, at the end of a long hill that leads into the city, there is a runaway truck ramp designed for vehicles that lose their brakes. I saw an eighteen-wheeler with a full load stuck in the loose, deep gravel, and oddly enough the scene reminded me of myself. Sometimes I just get moving too fast, carrying too heavy a load, and I end up stuck, unable to move. I know the problem: I take on a few too many projects. I bite off a little bit more than I can chew and end up yelling, "Lord! Where are You? I'm getting crushed with this load!" Then He gently reminds me that I proudly took the load upon myself. His yoke is easy; His load is light. I need to humble myself before God and admit my error. How can this be done? Verse 7 of 1 Peter 5 says, "Casting all your cares upon Him; for he careth for you" (KJV). I humble myself by admitting that I cannot handle the load I've put on myself, while speeding down the road of life. I've got to cast my cares, my burdens, my worries on the Lord, because He cares for me!

Prayer starter: Lord, as I prepare to become a mother, You know the pressures I feel. I cast these cares on You and pray for Your guidance and wisdom.

DAY

36

"One of the soldiers pierced Jesus' side with a spear, bringing a sudden flow of blood and water" *(John 19:34).*

Candy, a friend of mine who is the mother of four, told me that while she was pregnant with her first child she asked the Lord, "How can You know what I'll go through to give birth? When You walked the earth, You came in a man's body." Candy said the Lord answered her by saying that through His death upon the cross, as a result of shedding of His blood and water, the church was born. He understands the process of birth; He designed it.

Prayer starter: Lord, I thank and praise You once again that through the shed blood of Jesus Christ I can have new life. I pray for this baby I'm carrying that at the earliest possible moment she will come to know Jesus Christ as Lord and Savior.

DAY 37

"The body is a unit, though it is made up of many parts; and though all its parts are many, they form one body. So it is with Christ. For we were all baptized by one Spirit into one body" *(1 Cor. 12:12-13).*

Thom recently took our three-year-old David into the men's room at a restaurant. With all the stalls taken, Thom lifted little David so that he could utilize the urinal on the wall. As he accomplished his task from his father's arms, David announced loudly to the crowd in the men's room, "Now that's what I call cooperation!"

Even a small child can understand that people working together can do more than one person can hope to accomplish alone. Just as one's physical body has many members that allow it to function, so the body of Christ has a diversity of members who need to cooperate in unity and love in order for God's purposes to be accomplished.

Prayer starter: Father, show me the special place You have for me in Your body, so that I might be able to serve You and my brothers and sisters in Christ to the very best of my ability. Bless my baby with special giftings, so that he, too, will have a unique work to perform in Your kingdom.

DAY 38

"So do not fear, for I am with you; do not be dismayed, for I am your God. I will strengthen you and help you; I will uphold you with my righteous right hand" *(Is. 41:10).*

"Have you ever been scared, Mom?" Holly asked out of the blue.
"Yes, honey. Do you mean as a child or as a grown-up?"
"As a grown-up."
"Yes, I was scared when I went to the hospital to have Benjamin,

but God was with me, and pretty soon I wasn't scared anymore.''

"Were you scared when I didn't get off the school bus?'' she asked me softly, referring to an incident that had happened months earlier, an incident that she had not wanted to discuss with me.

The kindergarten school bus driver had not noticed that she was on the bus and skipped her stop. Afraid to say anything, she rode with him until the very end of the line. In the meantime, I called the school to see where the bus was and for about fifteen minutes had the teachers and principal frantically searching the halls for my missing daughter. When she and the school bus supervisor pulled up to my house in a van, I ran out to get her, crying and thanking God for her safety. The supervisor didn't say much, and Holly wouldn't tell me what happened until now.

"Were you afraid?'' I asked.

She nodded slowly, tears welling in her eyes.

I gave her a big hug. "Whenever you're afraid, you can pray and ask God to help you. He won't ever leave you.''

Prayer starter: Father, help me to know that You never leave nor forsake me. Help me to teach my children to put their trust in You. I pray that if the little one I'm carrying ever gets scared You will comfort her and give her Your peace.

DAY 39

"Listen to advice and accept instruction, and in the end you will be wise" *(Prov. 19:20).*

When I was pregnant with Holly, many women gave me advice. The instruction that lined up with God's Word proved to be very helpful to me throughout pregnancy and into new motherhood. At a shower given by the women in my church, I received informative books on child care and breast-feeding. The gifts that were foreign to me, like lap pads and snapping T-shirts, were explained.

One trusted friend, who is a little older and the mother of four children, became my personal consultant for questions ranging from what kind of clothes to wear home from the hospital to taking a newborn baby's temperature and what to do when you know you've eaten something that gives your nursing baby gas pains. I've found her advice and that of a few wise older women enormously helpful.

Prayer starter: Lord, help me listen to advice and accept instruction from others. Give me discernment so that I can weigh the advice given and make the right decisions for my unique circumstances. Thank You for giving me godly, experienced friends who love me enough to offer advice.

DAY 40

"Pleasant words are as an honeycomb, sweet to the soul, and health to the bones" *(Prov. 16:24, KJV).*

"Shem, would you like some chocolate ice cream?" I overheard my very round friend Ellen asking her large belly. "Oh, you would? Great! I'd like some too."

"What are you doing? Who is Shem?" I asked.

"Well, since I don't know if this baby is a boy or a girl, I put 'she' and 'him' together and get 'Shem.' Then, when I have important decisions to make, I ask Shem first. It's really amazing how much we think alike already," Ellen said with a twinkle in her eye.

I think of Ellen when I'm feeling a little low, because she has such a joyful, bubbly sense of humor. "A merry heart doeth good like a medicine," Proverbs 17:22 says. The ability to laugh certainly helps me when my hormones seem to be saying, "Cry, cry!"

Prayer starter: Lord, help me to speak pleasant words to my baby even now, and help me after this child is born to continue to have a sense of humor.

DAY 41

"May the words of my mouth and the meditation of my heart be pleasing in your sight, O Lord, my Rock and my Redeemer" *(Ps. 19:14).*

"Wimp! You're a baby!" shouts one of the big kids on the playground.

"Sticks and stones will break my bones, but words will never hurt me!'' the little boy yells back with great satisfaction. We've all grown up hearing this statement, but it's not true. Sticks and stones can break bones, but words can break hearts. I've heard parents call their children ''our little accidents.'' This may seem cute and harmless on the surface, but those words plant seeds in the child's mind that perhaps he's unloved or unwanted. Whatever the unkind words, the enemy can use them for his evil purposes.

If you're experiencing an unplanned pregnancy, why not smile and consider your child a surprise gift from the Lord rather than an accident? ''The tongue has the power of life and death,'' Proverbs 18:21 says. Will you speak words of life or words of death to your baby?

Prayer starter: Lord, let my words be pleasing in Your eyes. Forgive me when I say things that tear others down rather than build them up. Bless this baby's lips and tongue as they form. Anoint them to speak words of life and love to his generation.

DAY 42

"Man shall not live by bread alone, but by every word that proceedeth out of the mouth of God" *(Matt. 4:4, KJV).*

For breakfast this morning I scrambled one egg with an ounce of tofu, placed this on a toasted bagel, and topped it with some shredded Swiss cheese and alfalfa sprouts. Yumm!

Just as a pregnant woman must carefully plan her meals, making sure she eats a good balance of protein, carbohydrates, fruits and vegetables, and dairy products, so must we as Christians get a well-balanced diet of God's Word. A few years ago Thom brought two copies of the *One-Year Bible* (Tyndale House Publishers) home. We decided to read through the Bible together, one day at a time, using the arrangement in this book. Every day we read passages from the Old and New Testaments, the Psalms and Proverbs. After their bedtime stories, I try to read a section to the children and talk to them about what it means. The result is that we adults are getting a well-balanced diet of the Word of God. The children receive a taste of it, too!

Prayer starter: Lord, help me to feast on Your Word daily, nourishing my spirit with the bread of life. Help me to instill in my children the importance of reading Your Word. I pray that, as early as the child I'm carrying can hear, he, too, will have his spirit fed by Your Word as I read it out loud.

DAY 43

"Grandchildren are the crown of old men" (*Prov. 17:6, NAS*).

This baby is my parents' eighth grandchild and Thom's parents' fourth. With one of my sisters and Thom's sister also pregnant, these sets of grandparents are expecting numbers nine and five. Both sets of parents shower love, attention and concern on our children. All four grandparents are armed with plenty of photographs of grandchildren which they're ready and willing to display at the drop of a hat. We're so thankful to have wonderful grandparents for our children!

My heart goes out to those whose parents and grandparents are gone or live far away or for some reason or another are unable to participate in the lives of their grandchildren. God knows how important the extended family is, and He enables, through the church, even orphans to have parents and grandparents. If your baby needs a grandmother or grandfather, look in your local church body for a person or couple who may be willing to be an adopted grandparent. The wisdom of another generation will enrich you and your child, and the sense of need and love could enrich the adopted grandparent's life as well.

Prayer starter: Lord, thank You for creating the family. I pray for my extended family that each member will be supportive, loving and encouraging to this new baby as she grows. Be with all the expectant moms who do not have their own mothers and grandmothers with them to share this special time in their lives. Help them to find special relationships through Your body.

DAY 44

"And if the Spirit of him who raised Jesus from the dead is living in you, he who raised Christ from the dead will also give life to your mortal bodies through his Spirit, who lives in you" *(Rom. 8:11).*

If the Spirit that raised Jesus Christ from the dead is able to give life to our mortal bodies, He can also give life to the little body that is growing inside of us. Put your hand on your belly each day and pray to God that His Spirit will bless your child's rapidly growing body—cell by cell, bone by bone, every nerve, muscle, tissue, hair and tooth.

Prayer starter: Father, from the top of her head, to the tip of her toe, I pray in Jesus' name that You will bless this baby and cause her to form perfectly according to Your design.

DAY 45

"May your father and mother be glad; may she who gave you birth rejoice!" *(Prov. 23:25).*

Thom and I gathered the children around the dinner table to tell them about their new sibling.

"Holly, David and Benjamin, Daddy and I have something very important to tell you," I announced.

Thom continued, "Mommy and I are praising the Lord because He's giving us another child. A baby is growing in Mommy's tummy. It's very tiny now, but in a long while, you'll have another brother or sister," Thom tenderly told the children.

Holly grinned from ear to ear and said, "I hope it's a girl."

"The Lord knows what's best for our family. He gave us each of you," I said. "We don't know if this baby is a boy or a girl, but whatever it is, we're going to love this baby, just as we love each one of you."

Benjamin, at twenty months, didn't have much to say. He just sat in his high chair smiling at the air of excitement in the room.

David, three, contemplated all that was said, then asked very seriously, "Will the new baby poop yellow?"

No amount of parental training can provide an answer to a question like this. We squelched our laughter and simply said, "Yes, David, that's what little babies do."

"I know that, Daddy," David said. "Kori's new sister poops yellow. Kori told me so in Sunday school."

I'm sure our church's education department would be pleased to know the biblical truths that our children learn and share during class.

Prayer starter: Lord, we're glad! We rejoice already with the news of this new baby. I ask in Jesus' name that this child bring joy to my husband and me and to his brothers and sisters in the family here and in the family of God.

DAY 46

"He is like a tree planted by streams of water, which yields its fruit in season and whose leaf does not wither. Whatever he does prospers" *(Ps. 1:3).*

Picture a balmy palm tree growing on the bank of a desert stream. Because of the water, the tree grows, producing fruit that will in turn nourish others. I have a river of life literally flowing inside of me! My baby is growing in a sack of water. As this child feeds upon God's Word, seasoned with prayer, covered with love and anointed with God's Holy Spirit, she will produce fruit to feed her generation, giving life to all around her.

Prayer starter: Lord, I praise You, I thank You and I love You for Your eternal stream of living water. Please nourish this seedling of mine into a tree of righteousness. Give me eternal eyes to raise this baby to serve You forever and ever.

DAY 47

"From the lips of children and infants you have ordained praise" *(Matt. 21:16).* **"Thou has made children and babes at the breast sound aloud thy praise"** *(NEB).*

53

With big smiles and happy giggles the babies in our church nursery raise their hands when I say, "Praise the Lord!" Before their mouths form recognizable words, these babies can sing and praise God.

I remember when David was two we were traveling in the car with the whole family. David was drifting to sleep late at night as we crossed the Ohio River and entered Cincinnati. With the lights of the city glowing, David looked out the window and sang softly, "Let everything I do bring glory to Your name," a little praise chorus Thom wrote. David sang the song over and over again, mispronouncing the word "glory," singing "gwowy" instead. Thom and I looked at each other with praise and thanksgiving to God as we heard that baby voice sing praises to God.

Prayer starter: O Father, I pray this baby has a heart to praise and worship You. Even within the womb, let him hear me singing of You.

DAY
48
"The Lord saveth not with sword and spear: for the battle is the Lord's, and he will give you into our hands" *(1 Sam. 17:47, KJV).*

My uncle recently sang to my children a song that was popular during World War I: "America, I raised a boy for you...." The boy goes off to fight for his country, then his mother sings, "And if I had another, he'd march beside his brother. America, here's my boy." Uncle Bill said his grandmother used to cry when she heard the song, and for good reason. During her life she bore twelve children, including my grandfather, who fought in World Wars I and II.

The song brought tears to my eyes, too, thinking of my two toddling sons. I pray their world will know peace, so that they'll never have to march off to war.

A war is being waged between God and His enemies. As a mother I have a job to equip my sons and daughters with the weapons of this warfare. This battle isn't fought with spears, swords, missiles or bombs. It's fought with prayer, love, the preaching of God's Word and praise. By training our children to fight in the Lord's army, we prepare them for the only war that will matter in eternity.

Prayer starter: Lord, I pray my children will grow in a world that knows peace. I vow to train this baby in Your ways, Father, so that he will be a warrior for You.

DAY 49

"...beauty for ashes, the oil of joy for mourning, the garment of praise for the spirit of heaviness" *(Is. 61:3, KJV).*

When our children cry or whine unnecessarily, Thom pulls out his "magic" handkerchief, places it over the pouting face and announces he is going to turn a frown into a smile. He lifts the handkerchief with a loud "tuh-duh!" Sure enough, a smile appears.

As adults, when we're feeling low, we can choose to put on a "garment of praise for the spirit of heaviness." At first, this act is much like Thom's handkerchief. Praising God can be a willful decision. But when we focus on God, a miracle can occur. God does indeed dwell in our praise. His peace fills our hearts; His joy rejuvenates our heavy spirits.

Prayer starter: Lord, some days I feel so blue. I don't feel at all like worshipping You. I get tired and irritable. But, Father, I love You, and I thank You most of all for who You are, my loving Daddy. Thank You that because of Jesus I'll be able to spend eternity singing and shouting praise to You.

DAY 50

"It is of the Lord's mercies that we are not consumed, because his compassions fail not. They are new every morning" *(Lam. 3:22-23, KJV).*

When Thom and I were married, we moved into his apartment inside WPLW radio, a Christian station Thom managed. Because my training had been in journalism, I was picked to be the news department. Each morning I'd rise around 5:00 a.m., climb down the ladder from our bedroom into the first floor of the station, turn on the transmitter, then gather information for the first newscast at 6:00 a.m. I'd tear the copy from the wire service machines, get the weather forecast and traffic report, then type the headlines. Since many of our listeners set their alarms to awaken when WPLW signed on the air, I tried my best to help start people on the right foot. News of car wrecks and thunderstorms doesn't usually inspire people. I'd search for ''good news'' features to share what God and His church were doing in our community, and I'd select Scripture passages to remind people that God's mercies are ''new every morning.''

I think I'm better at helping others rise pleasantly than doing so myself. Especially now when I don't feel well, it's hard for me to get up in the morning thinking about singing. Nonetheless, God's mercy does not fail, and morning is a good time to get alone with Him and start the day right.

Prayer starter: Lord, thank You for another day and for Your love and compassion. Help me to awaken each day giving thanks and praise to You. I pray my baby will also awaken happily, praising You for health and strength.

DAY 51

"I pursued my enemies and overtook them; I did not turn back till they were destroyed. I crushed them so that they could not rise; they fell beneath my feet" *(Ps. 18:37-38).*

Pregnancy gives me added incentive to develop good habits and to eliminate bad ones. Proper diet and exercise will benefit mother and baby alike. My bad habits likewise affect my baby as well as myself. Now is a good time to say no once and for all to poor eating and sleeping habits. Those who smoke or are addicted to caffeine or any other drug or alcohol need to crush these enemies and not ever look back to them again.

Prayer starter: Lord, You know my faults and shortcomings better than I know them myself. I confess my bad habits and pray that You'll give me Your strength to overcome them. Bless my baby with good health. Please bless the nutrients that the baby receives and cause them to bring health and strength to my growing child.

DAY 52

"Whatsoever thy hand findeth to do, do it with thy might" *(Eccl. 9:10).*

It hasn't been too long since Benjamin was a tiny baby. I can remember him at four months playing with a piece of paper. His uncoordinated little hands would flail wildly at the paper until he grabbed hold of it. Then he would shake it with all his might and giggle at the sound of the paper crumpling in his pudgy fist. His whole being seemed to be wrapped up in this playful activity.

I need to be reminded to complete each task I attempt with the enthusiasm Benjamin poured into his paper game. Sometimes I think I need blinders—like those that horses wear to prevent distractions—from pulling me off course. I'm particularly tired right now, so I need more willpower than ever to accomplish the tasks of the day.

Prayer starter: Father, help me this day to have a clear idea of my priorities, then to accomplish each task, whether boring or exciting, to the best of my ability. I pray that You will bless my baby's little hands even as they are forming. Help this child, as he grows older, to use his hands mightily to do Your will.

DAY 53

"The Lord was with Joseph and he prospered, and he lived in the house of his Egyptian master. When his master saw that the Lord was with him and that the Lord gave him success in everything he did, Joseph found favor in his eyes and became his attendant" *(Gen. 39:2).*

Egypt in Scripture represents the world outside of God's kingdom. In living with the Egyptians, Joseph was surrounded by people who did not know God. Yet the Bible says of him, "The Lord gave him success in everything he did." Because of his accomplishments, the Egyptian master blessed Joseph.

As a mother, I can think of no greater hope and prayer for my children. First, I pray that they know God; second, that God will bless them; and third, that instead of the world's beating them down, they will find success and favor in the eyes of others.

Prayer starter: Lord, I thank You for the example of Joseph and how he overcame adversity to be a blessing to both his own people and the entire world. I pray that You will bless the child within me with success in his endeavors and favor both in Your eyes and in the eyes of the world.

DAY 54

"But the very hairs of your head are all numbered" *(Matt. 10:30, KJV).*

One of my sisters told me that while she carried her two children, she and her husband affectionately referred to the babies as Bozo and Bozette. I inherited my mother's tradition of referring to the baby as Oscar. (Thom invented the feminine form of Oscarina.) My sister who is pregnant now refers to her baby with the neutral name Flash.

It's so hard to imagine what this little baby's name should be, when we don't know if it's a boy or a girl. We don't know the color of the baby's hair or eyes. Thom and I have difficulty in narrowing our name choices down to a final selection for male and female.

But even though we earthly parents have trouble in deciding on a name for our child, our heavenly Father knows and loves the baby intimately. He's forming each part of the child and even has numbered the hairs on his head. Sometimes I wish I could get a glimpse of this baby through the Lord's eyes.

Prayer starter: Father, I'm thankful once again that You're blessing me with this baby. I know that no matter how much I love this child You love him more and know what's best for him. Give me Your eyes to see and Your ears to hear so that I'll become a godly mother, carved in Your image.

DAY

55

"The midwives answered Pharaoh, 'Hebrew women are not like Egyptian women; they are vigorous and give birth before the midwives arrive' " *(Ex. 1:19).*

Be careful how you pray! When I was eight months pregnant with David, a woman asked if she could pray for me and my baby. I said, "Sure." Then she prayed diligently, "Father, I pray that this child will be born quickly and easily, and that, just like the Hebrew women, Cathy will have this baby before there's time for the midwife to arrive."

About a month later, I awoke feeling a little funny. With no contractions or other signs of labor, I thought I might have had a touch of the flu. I felt a little crampy, so I called the doctor and he said to come to the hospital. On the way to the hospital, I had a very serious contraction; I felt like pushing. I didn't know what to do but pray: "Lord, I'd really prefer to have this baby in the hospital instead of the car. Please help us get there!"

Outside the hospital doors in the parking lot, I had to breathe through another very effective contraction. At the admission desk, I calmly told the nurse I thought I was in very active labor. She stared at me with a "Yeah, sure" attitude. Then I had another contraction. I sat on the floor and started breathing deeply.

Within seconds I was placed on a bed and wheeled to the labor suite. Several nurses undressed me, as I heard my doctor's name paged over the public address system. We went straight to the delivery room where one of the nurses confirmed what we all knew: the baby was crowning and ready to be born!

The nurse said, "Please try to blow through your next contraction. We know how to deliver a baby, but we'd really like to wait for the doctor." I heard another doctor being summoned to the delivery room as the next contraction came.

If the nurse wants to wait for the doctor, then so do I, I thought, as I breathed deeply through the next contraction. To my joy, both Thom and my own doctor suddenly appeared.

"Go ahead and push on the next contraction," my doctor said.

David was born, screaming loudly, on that next contraction. Thom got a photograph, and all the nurses cheered. The time was 9:52 a.m.

It hadn't even been an hour since we left the house! David came very quickly, with barely enough time for the doctor to arrive.

Prayer starter: Father, I pray that You will bless the delivery of this baby I'm carrying. I pray for a quick and easy delivery, but I'd really prefer to have my health-care worker present and for there to be plenty of time to prepare for the actual birth of this baby.

DAY 56

"Like newborn babies, crave pure spiritual milk, so that by it you may grow up in your salvation, now that you have tasted that the Lord is good" *(1 Pet. 2:2-3).*

One of the wonders of childbirth occurs when a wailing newborn is placed on a woman's belly and she puts the child to her breast. A God-given instinct causes that baby to suck hungrily, unless he is drowsy from drugs or anesthetics the mother took during labor. The first milk a newborn receives, called colostrum, provides precious natural immunities against disease. Then from two to six days after delivery (with me it was the third day), a mother's milk comes in.

When my Benjamin, who already had a strong sucking instinct, tasted "real" milk, he acted like a little piglet who had been treated with a feast. Even after his newborn stage, he nursed so loudly that I couldn't sit in church feeding him discreetly as I had with Holly and David. His loud gulping noises disturbed the people sitting around me.

Just as a newborn craves his mother's milk, Peter admonishes us to hunger for God's Word. I like to think of Benjamin's sweet little face, as he gulped away, when I read this verse. Do I have that kind of appetite for my Bible reading? Hmmm. Benjamin has grown from an infant into a sturdy toddler. If I'm to grow spiritually, I must crave and feed upon God's Word.

Prayer starter: Lord, thank You for speaking to me through Your Word. Thank You for feeding my spirit, helping me to mature in my faith. I pray that the child within me will be born with a strong, healthy urge to eat and that as she grows she will also crave spiritual food.

DAY 57

"Yet you brought me out of the womb; you made me trust in you even at my mother's breast" *(Ps. 22:9).*

When I meditate upon this verse, I can envision the Lord gently delivering my baby. His hands offer a blessing and anointing at this child's birth. His Spirit rests upon the baby from his first breath, wooing the child to follow Him.

This verse also assures me that the baby will not be born too early or too late. If God Himself brings him out of the womb, the timing will be perfect.

Prayer starter: Father, thank You for Your Word and the examples in it that I can cling to and meditate upon. I trust You to deliver this child, to bring him out of my womb when the time is right. I pray that he will trust in You from his first breath.

DAY 58

"As a mother comforts her child, so will I comfort you" *(Is. 66:13).*

Benjamin stood on his high chair, and before I had the chance to grab him, he fell, pulling the chair on top of him. The chair split his lip open, so I rushed him to the medical center close to our house. Clinging to me in pain and fear, Benjamin sobbed while the doctor tried to examine him. He needed a few stitches, so two nurses peeled little Ben away from me and took him screaming and kicking into the treatment area. Everyone in the waiting room could hear his cries as the lip was stitched. I knew the injury was minor, but the intense sorrow in Benjamin's voice cut into my heart. I wanted to sit down and cry, but I didn't.

When the doctor was finished, Benjamin ran out into the waiting room to me. I scooped him into my arms and tried to comfort him, singing softly in his ear, telling him what a big boy he was and how much I loved him. In a few minutes the sobs and cries stopped, and he lay his head on my shoulder.

We often think of God as Father, but Scripture compares the Lord to a loving mother as well. When we're hurt, in pain, fearful and out of control, God comforts us as we mothers would comfort our child. When we turn to God for help, He wraps His arms of love around us and whispers, "Don't be afraid. I love you. I'm always here for you." Just as Benjamin stopped crying and rested on my shoulder, we can find peace and rest in the Lord.

Prayer starter: Lord, thank You for Your unfailing love. I thank You that when I'm hurt or afraid, I can come to You. I pray that You'll protect my little child from harm, but when the bumps and bruises of life come, help me to follow Your example so that I can be a loving, comforting parent.

DAY 59

"Let the saints rejoice in this honor and sing for joy on their beds" *(Ps. 149:5).*

Lying on my bed this morning, it takes all the energy I have to turn around to grab the tasteless wheat crackers that are ready for me on the shelf. Eating a cracker while my head is still down helps my stomach to settle just a bit.

"Lord, bless this cracker and help it to stay down."

Why do you suppose there is a Scripture verse that says, "Let the saints sing for joy on their beds"? Surely God knew there would be days like today, when I don't feel like opening my eyes, let alone singing and dancing and going on with the challenge of a new morning.

Yet, despite how I feel, I can rejoice. I will sing for joy on my bed, because God is good. He's blessing me with new life. Morning sickness may be from the pit of hell, but Satan will not rob me of my joy in Jesus.

Prayer starter: Lord, I praise and thank You for another new day. I pray You'll touch my body, strengthen me, help every part of me to function the way You intended. Bless this baby, and please allow him to be properly nourished even when I don't feel well.

What thoughts have you had this month? How do you feel? How much weight have you gained? If you've been to the doctor, what did he or she say? Have any special Scripture verses or meditations ministered to you this month? Have you been praying for God to bless the fruit of joy in your life? Have you seen results?

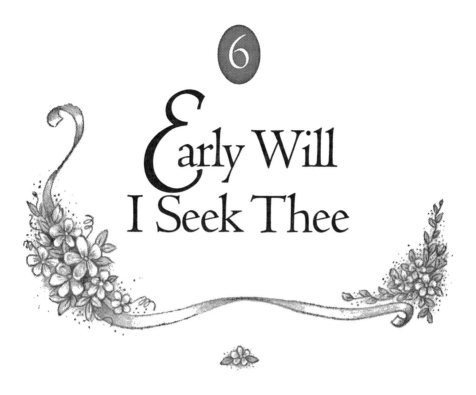

6

$\mathcal{E}$arly Will I Seek Thee

D A Y S   6 0 – 8 9

MONTH THREE

During this month the baby will grow to three inches and weigh about one ounce. Did you ever see the tiny feet that pro-life advocates wear on their lapels? These feet are the size of your baby at ten weeks. Even at this early stage in development the child looks like a miniature person, complete with beautifully formed feet. During this month the baby will begin to open and close its mouth, swallowing amniotic fluid. The kidneys will function, and the baby will be able to move its limbs, although you won't feel that movement yet. Nails and teeth develop, earlobes form and eyes are almost complete. The baby's heartbeat can be heard with special instruments. Reproductive organs are developing, although it is difficult to determine the baby's sex.

You may or may not finally "feel" pregnant. It is not unusual to experience nausea, frequent urination, heartburn, fatigue, constipation, tenderness in your breasts, and food cravings. You may notice your veins looking large and blue as your blood supply increases. Some people never have any of these symptoms; some may have one or two. However you feel, be sure to get plenty of rest, eat nutritious food and drink plenty of water. If you have been feeling very sick and tired, be of good cheer. By the end of the third month, most people (including me) feel better as their bodies adjust to the pregnant state.

Prayer starter: Father, bless my baby and all the developing organs. I pray that every physical aspect of this child's body will be formed perfectly according to Your plan.

DAY 60

"O God, thou art my God; early will I seek thee: my soul thirsteth for thee, my flesh longeth for thee in a dry and thirsty land, where no water is" *(Ps. 63:1, KJV).*

A soft orange light glows on the eastern horizon. Out my window I can see a flock of birds resting on telephone wires. Their morning song greets the sun, chirping away the pre-dawn darkness. The robins and sparrows praise the Lord, but I can't get my head off the pillow. When will my stomach settle down? Will my head ever stop spinning? Soda crackers and water help the nausea a little. Eating protein, like peanut butter on wheat toast before I go to bed, helps a little more because the food is digested slowly, releasing nutrients over the long hours between dinner and breakfast. Last night I didn't feel like eating a peanut butter sandwich as a bedtime snack, but this morning I wish I had.

I know this nausea will cease, and I look forward to the day when I hold my baby and praise the Lord that all went well.

Prayer starter: O God, I need You early this morning! Help me know what to do to settle my stomach without getting sick. I pray my baby will be safe, even if I can't hold down breakfast. Yet even while my body aches, my soul hungers and thirsts for You, Lord; I know You satisfy my needs.

DAY
61 "The fruit of the Spirit is...peace" *(Gal. 5:22).*

To bear the fruit of peace, we must first be sure that we're at peace with God and not His enemy. Romans 5:10 says, "For if, when we were enemies, we were reconciled to God by the death of his Son..." (KJV). Are you reconciled to God through Christ Jesus? If the answer is yes, then you can be at peace with God. Since God has forgiven you, you can likewise forgive all who hurt you, allowing you to live in peace with *every* person on the face of the earth, including your unborn child.

The inner peace we have, knowing that we're children of God, gives us the ability to live peaceful lives, even amidst strife, battles, bickerings and fights. We don't have to fight to hold on to our own little turf if our lives are built on the rock, Jesus Christ. We need not be defensive or quarrelsome when Christ is our cornerstone.

He told His disciples in John 14:27: "Peace I leave with you; my peace I give you. I do not give to you as the world gives. Do not let your hearts be troubled and do not be afraid" (NIV). Did you hear that? Even if a nuclear war erupts right outside your door, your soul can have peace in Christ.

If our hearts are at peace, our actions will be as well. During this third month of pregnancy most abortions take place. Abortion is a violent way to deal with a perceived conflict. Christ's peace is life-giving, both to the body and the spirit.

Prayer starter: Lord, sow Your peace into my life. As Saint Francis wrote, "Make me an instrument of Your peace" to the world around me. I pray for the mothers of unborn babies, who are in their third month of pregnancy. Bless us all with a spirit of peace. Protect the innocent. Fill my baby with Your peace that passes understanding.

DAY
62 "And if the Spirit of him who raised Jesus from the dead is living in you, he who raised Christ from the dead will also give life" *(Rom. 8:11).*

"I can't do it! I can't have a baby," a friend sobbed. "I'm too scared!"

Her husband was saddened and prayed God would change her mind and give her peace about having children. They'd been married several years and he very much wanted to be a father. My friend wanted children, too, but she could not get over this fear of childbirth.

If you're having similar fears about childbirth, know that God gives us the power to do whatever He wants us to do. Clearly, if God put the desire in a woman's heart to bear a child, He is able to empower her to succeed.

God told Moses to raise his staff, and the Red Sea became a road to freedom. He led Daniel into the den of hungry lions and sent an angel to "shut the mouths of the lions." He told a young virgin named Mary that she was pregnant with His Son, then gave her the power to receive the news rejoicing!

We can have the power to do anything God wills through the same Spirit that raised Christ from the dead. We need not fear bearing children. We do so by God's design; He'll give us the wisdom, strength and courage we need.

My friend, after a long period of asking God to remove her fear, became pregnant. Full of faith, she prayed and praised God along with her husband for nine months. She read, exercised and resisted Satan when he came to harass her with thoughts of fear. Just recently, I heard the news that she gave birth to a nine-pound, beautiful, blond baby boy. Praise God! Her delivery was smooth and quick. She did not succumb to fear.

Prayer starter: Lord, thank You for making Your Holy Spirit available to empower me to do Your will. Fill me with Your Spirit, so that I can have Your strength to carry this baby to term and deliver him safely.

DAY
63

"For the word of God is living and active. Sharper than any double-edged sword, it penetrates even to dividing soul and spirit, joints and marrow; it judges the thoughts and attitudes of the heart" *(Heb. 4:12).*

When we read the Bible, we give God the opportunity to slash through our exterior walls and pierce our underlying thoughts. When the Word is read aloud, this power is released to do God's work in all who hear it. The Amplified Bible further illuminates this verse by saying, "For the Word that God speaks is alive and full of power—making it active, operative, energizing and effective; it is sharper than any two-edged sword, penetrating to the dividing line of the breath of life (soul) and [the immortal] spirit, and of joints and marrow [that is, of the deepest parts of our nature] exposing and sifting and analyzing and judging the very thoughts and purposes of the heart."

I honestly do not know when the unborn child begins to hear. As early as twenty-four weeks some babies have responded to sound, and most can hear by thirty weeks (*Hippocrates*, Keiko Ohnuma, July/August 1987). I don't think it's ever too early to read the Bible out loud to your child. The experience will set a pattern for you to follow when the child begins to hear. It could also build your faith, for the Bible says, "Faith comes from hearing the message, and the message is heard through the word of Christ" (Rom. 10:17).

Prayer starter: Lord, help me to be diligent in reading Your Word. I pray it cuts through the garbage in my life, bringing Your power to everything I think and do. I pray for my baby that Your Word will bring life, health and strength to her bones, joints and marrow, even as her body is forming.

DAY 64

"Let him kiss me with the kisses of his mouth—for your love is more delightful than wine" *(Song 1:2).*

One of our single friends came for dinner recently. When we told him I was pregnant again, he voiced a concern to Thom that astounded me. He hoped and prayed Thom wouldn't turn elsewhere for sexual gratification, assuming couples did not make love during a woman's pregnancy. Counting one miscarriage, this is my fifth pregnancy in six years. Our friend thought we were practically celibate!

I assure you, such is not the case. Although I believe you should follow your own doctor's guidelines, there is no need for abstinence from sexual relations during a healthy pregnancy. In their classic

Christian book *Intended for Pleasure* (Revell) Ed and Gaye Wheat say, "Physicians have been in general agreement that intercourse during pregnancy uncomplicated by bleeding or episodes of premature labor or a history of high-risk pregnancy should be safe enough, at least during the first eight months."

The husband, say the Wheats, "should be even more affectionate and complimentary than usual. Treating her with tenderness and appreciation during pregnancy will pay great dividends in sexual pleasure for both partners, and will have lasting benefits." And for the wife: "Psychologically, your husband needs to feel an emotional bond with you and his baby...he needs to be reassured that he has not permanently exchanged his lover/companion for someone interested only in motherhood. Remember that although pregnancy may change your sexual desires, your husband is not pregnant. His sexual needs continue at the same level throughout the pregnancy, delivery, and the weeks of abstention afterward."

This book discusses the subject of sex during pregnancy at great length. I highly recommend that both husband and wife read it.

Prayer starter: Lord, I pray for my husband that during this time of pregnancy his affection will grow and our relationship deepen. I pray we both will be open and honest concerning our sexual needs and that we'll both be sensitive to the needs of the other.

DAY
65

"We take captive every thought to make it obedient to Christ" *(2 Cor. 10:5).*

Think lovely things. If an ugly, un-Christlike thought enters your mind, the Bible says to "demolish arguments and every pretension that sets itself up against the knowledge of God." If your greatest fear is that the baby will be unhealthy in some way, pray for your child, speak words of health and strength to him. Be educated concerning the incidence of birth defects. Avoid practices that are known to contribute to problems for the baby. After you've made sure that what you do is good for the baby, and you're praying and reading your Bible, deal with your negative thoughts. Don't ignore them, because they won't go away. The Bible says to take each thought captive. In Philippians 4:8 the apostle Paul tells us to let our minds dwell on things that are pure and lovely, excellent and praiseworthy. Compare your thoughts to your knowledge of God, then eliminate anything that is ungodly.

Prayer starter: Father, I acknowledge my negative thoughts and fears and ask Your forgiveness for them. I know that Your perfect love casts out fear, so I receive Your love and freedom from fear. You know my concerns about the health of this child. I vow to do my best to care for this baby, to eat, drink and care for my body wisely. After that, I gladly commit my life and my child's life into Your hands anew.

DAY
66

"Who is a God like you, who pardons sin and forgives the transgression of the remnant of his inheritance? You do not stay angry forever but delight to show mercy. You will again have compassion on us; you will tread our sins underfoot and hurl all our iniquities into the depths of the sea" *(Mic. 7:18-19).*

Thom and I have made a deal for this pregnancy. From past experience, we know that changing hormone levels and fatigue wreak havoc on my normally even-tempered disposition. He has agreed to be very, very nice to me until the baby is six months old, when he'll continue to be just nice.

Today I know I blew it. We had an argument over something silly and I really became upset, crying, pouting, generally throwing an adult sort of tantrum. I know I was wrong for how I behaved, pregnant or not, so I must muster up the courage to apologize. Fortunately I not only have a God who loves and forgives me when I make stupid errors, but I also have a godly husband who I know will also forgive me.

Prayer starter: Lord, thank You for Your forgiveness of sins. I ask You to pour Your mercy out on me. Forgive me when I allow my emotions to go out of control. I invite You to examine my heart further and show me the root of my error.

DAY

67

"Verily I say unto you, Among them that are born of women there hath not risen a greater than John the Baptist: notwithstanding he that is least in the kingdom of heaven is greater than he" *(Matt. 11:11, KJV)*.

What will this baby be like? Where will he go to school? What profession will he choose? Will he marry and have children? Will he make an impact on his generation? Will he be outgoing or shy?

Jesus said that John the Baptist was the greatest man ever born. John's task on earth was to tell mankind to prepare for the coming of the kingdom of God. "Repent ye: for the kingdom of heaven is at hand," he told the people.

Jesus Christ made the kingdom of God available to every person, becoming a sacrifice for all of our sins. When we repent, acknowledging Jesus as our Lord and Savior, we enter into the kingdom of God.

We mothers can follow in the footsteps of John the Baptist, crying, "Prepare ye the way of the Lord; make his paths straight" to our children.

If we truly want our sons and daughters to be great, we'll help prepare their hearts to accept Jesus Christ. Then, whether they choose to be teachers, doctors, homemakers or lion tamers, they'll be even greater than John the Baptist, according to Scripture, because they'll be citizens of heaven.

Prayer starter: Lord, I pray that this baby will have a heart to learn about You and to receive the good news that Jesus came to earth to die for all of our sins. Help me let the resurrection of Christ be evident in my life, so that my child will see You working through me. Whatever profession, personality type or appearance my child possesses, my constant prayer is that he enter into Your kingdom.

DAY

68

"Thou art my hiding place; thou shalt preserve me from trouble; thou shalt compass me about with songs of deliverance" *(Ps. 32:7, KJV)*.

I grew up in a big old house that had many interesting hiding places. Sometimes I would imagine myself in eminent danger: lions coming to devour me (inspired by old Tarzan movies), a nuclear holocaust or a Nazi search for Anne Frank and her family. I'd plan an escape route to my safe hiding place, whether it was in the old coal cellar or underneath the toys in the toy box.

I'm grown up now, but I sometimes still become frightened, not from the fear of ravaging hungry lions or Nazi soldiers, but from the threat that everyday living in the United States brings to me and my family.

It is comforting to know that I can go to the Lord and be protected. "He shall cover thee with his feathers, and under his wings shalt thou trust" (Ps. 91:4, KJV). How can I be afraid?

If I fear for myself or my children, the delivery of this baby, or my family's future plans, I must run to my hiding place, find comfort and protection in the Lord, then venture out into the world again to proceed with life and the tasks He's given me.

Prayer starter: Father, thank You that in You I have a hiding place from my troubles and fears. Nourish me through Your Word. Shelter me under Your wings.

DAY 69

"Surely the churning of milk bringeth forth butter, and the wringing of the nose bringeth forth blood: so the forcing of wrath bringeth forth strife" *(Prov. 30:33, KJV).*

I'm on my way to do an interview, first thing in the morning. A man in the elevator is smoking, even though there's a No Smoking sign quite evident. What should I do? Force my wrath on this pleasant-looking businessman? Throw up on his three-piece, navy blue, pin-striped suit?

It's crowded. I'm hot. The elevator door opens. Whoosh! More people board and I'm stuck even closer to this lawbreaker. As the elevator continues its ascent, all of my breakfast rises in my throat. "OH! I'M GOING TO BE SICK!" I announce frantically, covering my mouth. As if their coats were made of steel and the elevator walls were magnets, my fellow passengers stick to the walls, leaving me alone in the middle of the elevator. Mr. Smoker throws his cigarette to the floor and says, "I hope the smoke didn't bother you."

Too sick to respond, I just force myself to smile. I wish I were wearing maternity clothes so this guy wouldn't think I was a wimp. But I guess I am a wimp. Not wanting to cause strife by confronting a stranger, I made myself sick. I wonder what Jesus would do in a situation like this?

Prayer starter: Lord, give me the mind of Christ. Help me to deal lovingly and righteously with my fellow human beings. You know if it were just I, I wouldn't care too much. But I am concerned for the health of this baby. Give me power by Your Spirit to deal boldly with situations that may jeopardize my child's development.

DAY 70

"Above all, love each other deeply, because love covers over a multitude of sins" *(1 Pet. 4:8).*

When I was a little girl, my mother didn't teach me how to knead bread, darn socks, beat a rug or care for a newborn. This by no means is an indictment of her parenting skills. She did teach me skills necessary for survival in suburban America during the second half of the twentieth century. I can find bargains at shopping malls, make sandwiches and vacuum a rug. Unlike the families of preceding generations, there weren't a dozen siblings who came after me, or the newborn babies of cousins close by. Even though I had a few babysitting jobs as a teenager, I don't remember ever changing a diaper before Holly was born. Don't laugh. I remember being somewhat concerned about diaper-changing techniques just a few short years ago.

The mistakes we parents make as a result of ignorance and inexperience can be covered, the Bible says, by love. We will make mistakes through our trials and errors. We ought to confess our faults to God and to our children. But rather than living in worry that our offspring will be irreparably damaged by our mistakes, we should live in victory knowing that God's love working through us can heal hurts, cover problems and generally compensate for our shortcomings.

Prayer starter: Lord, I confess my feelings of inadequacy in regard to parenting this child properly. Thank You for Your unfailing love and for the power Your love brings to my life. Fill me with love for this child. Help me to love him deeply, covering a multitude of problems and errors that I'll surely make.

DAY 71

"Consider the ravens: They do not sow or reap, they have no storeroom or barn; yet God feeds them. And how much more valuable you are than birds!" *(Luke 12:24).*

One of my acquaintances, responding to the news of my pregnancy, commented, "How can you afford another baby? Are you able to take care of the three you have?"

Thinking she may have been offensive (which she was) she added, "I'd have had more than one child, but we couldn't afford another. I don't know how you manage with three. What will you ever do with four?"

Come on, Cathy, think of something loving, kind, Christ-like and truthful to say.

"I don't know. I guess God knows I need to pray a lot," I told her, instead of delivering the sermon that was running through my mind.

The truth is, God does provide all of my needs according to His riches in glory by Christ Jesus. I view my children as gifts, blessings from God. Sometimes we don't quite seem to make ends meet. Other times we're blessed with an abundance. But my family is clothed and fed and very happy.

"And seek not ye what ye shall eat, or what ye shall drink, neither be ye of doubtful mind. For all these things do the nations of the world seek after: and your Father knoweth that ye have need of these things. But rather seek ye the kingdom of God; and all these things shall be added unto you" (Luke 12:29-31, KJV).

I don't need to covet sixty-dollar tennis shoes for my children or designer bibs for this baby. My priorities are in order when I seek first the kingdom of God. He will provide for this new child.

Prayer starter: Father, thank You for Your provision for my family. I praise You for Your blessings. Help my whole family to keep our priorities straight, putting You first in all things.

DAY 72

"Trust in the Lord with all your heart and lean not on your own understanding; in all your ways acknowledge him, and he will make your paths straight" *(Prov. 3:5).*

One of my pregnant friends, the mother of two small boys, just had a sonogram. She's relieved to know that apparently the baby is just fine, but she's also disappointed, because she discovered the baby is a boy.

"I've been crying ever since I found out. We wanted a girl so badly. Don't tell me to try again. Three kids are enough!"

I told her the first thought that entered my mind: "God must have given you a special gifting to raise boys. This child is fortunate to have a mom and dad who are by now very experienced in parenting boys."

She seemed to hear what I said, thanked me, and said I'd given her food for thought. Trust in God! He is forming a unique individual inside of you. He has a special plan for you and your child.

Prayer starter: Lord, I trust in You and acknowledge You alone as the giver of life. I may not understand all Your plans for me, but I trust You to make them and to give me the power by Your Spirit to follow the path You've set. I trust that the child I'm carrying is the sex, size, color and shape that You've designed for Your perfect plan. Help me to be a good mother, whatever this baby is like.

DAY 73

"Then you will know the truth and the truth will set you free" *(John 8:32).*

The summer of 1976 I worked in Washington, D.C., in a congressional office. On the Fourth of July, our nation's two hundredth birthday, I joined a few hundred thousand others for what was billed as the most spectacular fireworks display in history, with special effects from lasers. The fireworks were great, but as I watched I couldn't figure out what the lasers were doing. I assumed that they were somewhere in the snap, crackle and pop of the fireworks. It turned out the laser show was a dud. Something went wrong. The lasers didn't work. I didn't even know it, because I didn't know what to look for. Consequently, I didn't know what I was missing.

The same thing happened to me in my spiritual life. I thought I was free. I did what I wanted, when I wanted. I led an active life but always wondered, "Where are the lasers? Is this all there is?" Loving Christians prayed for me and gave me things like the Gospel of John and C.S. Lewis's *Mere Christianity* to read. After much seeking I found the love that only comes into a person's life when he or she knows Jesus Christ. Until I was set free, I didn't know I had been bound.

Prayer starter: Thank You, Lord, for Your love. Thank You for revealing Yourself to me and for setting me free from all the cares and concerns and sins of this world that had me bound. I pray for my child that she will know You from a very early age, that she'll be set free from sin.

DAY
74

"O Lord, our Lord, how majestic is your name in all the earth! You have set your glory above the heavens. From the lips of children and infants you have ordained praise..." *(Ps. 8:1-2).*

My children all love to sing. Holly's first and favorite song was "Jesus Loves Me," which she called "The Bible Tells Me So" when she was two. David's first song was "He Is the King of Kings." Benjamin probably began singing in tune earlier than the others. He can sing the "ABC Song" and "His Banner Over Me Is Love," and he can't quite talk yet!

When we're in the car, we take turns choosing songs then singing them. This may sound monotonous and dull, but there are no words to describe the thrill and excitement I feel as a parent when I hear the joyful singing of my children.

How much more our heavenly Father must appreciate the praise and worship we offer to Him. We are His children; I know it pleases God when we sing for Him.

Prayer starter: O Lord, how majestic is Your name! Thank You, Father, for music and for the ability to sing before You. Give me a pure heart to praise You. Bless this baby with a joyful spirit and a gift to sing.

DAY 75

"As thou knowest not what is the way of the spirit, nor how the bones do grow in the womb of her that is with child; even so thou knowest not the works of God who maketh all" *(Eccl. 11:5, KJV).*

A few years ago I had the opportunity to interview a famous musician/evangelist whom many would recognize from his records and television appearances. I asked him if he could give my radio audience advice on overcoming weaknesses in their lives. I was very impressed with his answer. He said, "I don't know. It's not an area I seem to have much success with."

He could have spouted off a number of religious platitudes to cover for the fact that he was having some problems in his own life. But he didn't; he was real with the people, and I think as a result of his honesty, many of my listeners were encouraged that they were not the only ones with problems.

The apostle Paul told the Corinthians, "We see through a glass darkly; but then face to face: now I know in part; but then shall I know even as also I am known."

I don't know how my baby's bones are growing inside my womb. I do not understand many things about the works of God. But I know He loves me and wants the best for me. I must put my faith and trust in Him concerning the mysteries of life, including childbirth.

Prayer starter: I confess that there is plenty I don't understand. Help me to be real with my child, to admit my shortcomings and to turn to You for help. You know the forming child within me. Bless this baby with Your wisdom even as his bones are growing.

DAY

76

"The seed on good soil stands for those with a noble and good heart, who hear the word, retain it, and by perseverance produce a crop" *(Luke 8:15)*.

In a few months when we have our babies, we will nurture them. We'll feed them and tend to their every need. With proper care our children will grow from helpless newborns to sturdy toddlers in a matter of months. As loving mothers we would not dream of neglecting the babies we've planned and prayed for!

Likewise, our faith must be tended and nurtured if it is to grow. In the parable of the sower, Jesus tells of the farmer who planted seed. Some fell on the path and were eaten by birds. Some fell on rocks and quickly sprouted in the shallow soil, but they withered because they had no roots. Other seeds were choked out by weeds and thorns.

The kind of faith that produces a crop is rooted in the Word of God. It's protected by a community of loving fellow workers that help keep away predators. Faith bears fruit when the cares and worries of this world have no opportunity to choke and destroy it.

Prayer starter: Lord, even as this baby is nurtured and grows from a seed into an adult, bless my faith to grow and mature. Help me to be diligent in reading Your Word and seeking fellowship in Your body. Give me strength to rise above the cares of this world.

DAY

77

"Blessed art thou among women, and blessed is the fruit of thy womb" *(Luke 1:42, KJV)*.

Elizabeth, six months pregnant, pronounced this blessing upon her cousin Mary who carried the Christ child in her womb. Mary acknowledged her blessing and privilege saying, "My soul doth magnify the Lord...for behold, from henceforth all generations shall call me blessed." Indeed, Mary was blessed—the woman chosen to bear the Savior of the world.

Although none of us is carrying the Messiah, I think we're heirs of Mary's legacy as pregnant women. We're blessed with the gift of life. God has entrusted us with one of His precious creations. Did you ever stop to think that the Son of God began life as a single cell that divided and grew in the womb of a woman? God became extremely vulnerable as He trusted Mary to care for this blessed child. What an awesome responsibility!

I believe God pours out special blessings on pregnant women. He could have sent His Son into the world in a different way. The Messiah could have been formed out of the dust like Adam. A stork could have delivered Jesus on Mary's doorstep. He could have appeared as a full-grown person one day in Nazareth. But instead, God Himself, the Word made flesh, Jesus, spent nine months in a woman's womb.

How privileged we are to bear children—to be God's instruments to bring new life into the world!

Prayer starter: Father, thank You for Your gift of life. Thank You for blessing the fruit of my womb. I'm amazed at the thought that Jesus Christ, my Savior, came into the world the same way I did and the same way my child will. Help me to treat life as a precious and holy gift to be cherished and loved.

DAY 78

"Pay attention and listen to the sayings of the wise; apply your heart to what I teach, for it is pleasing when you keep them in your heart and have all of them ready on your lips" *(Prov. 22:17-18).*

From the first day of first grade, I loved school. I loved to learn. I enjoyed school so much that for a long time after graduating from college, I missed the classroom atmosphere. I don't seem to have in my own power the discipline to force myself to learn as I did in school. I believe strongly that I must continue to learn and grow, absorbing the knowledge I have and applying it to my life. To do this, sometimes I have to put myself back in the classroom atmosphere. Here's what I do:

1. At church, I sit down front with a notebook and Bible. Under the pastor's nose it's hard to daydream. If I sit in the back, my mind sometimes wanders from the teaching.

2. I have the entire Bible on cassette tapes. When I'm too lazy to have daily devotions, I pop on a tape in my car, in the kitchen or in the laundry room and listen to the Word of God. It *never* ceases to amaze me what lessons I learn when hearing the Word.

3. I pray as David prayed several times in the Psalms: "Teach me Your ways, Lord." I want to have a heart open to the things of God. When I least expect it, God teaches me a lesson.

Prayer starter: Lord, there's so much to learn about You, and I'm continually wandering off the path You have for me. Help me to keep growing, keep going with You. With a baby coming, I feel the need even greater to learn Your ways. Let them sink into my heart, so that in due time, Your wisdom will be on my lips when my child needs help. Help me now to learn of You.

DAY
79   "Be kind and compassionate to one another" *(Eph. 4:32).*

There are many decisions to make concerning pregnancy and childbirth. Where should the baby be born? Hospital, home or birth center? What type of childbirth method is best for me and my baby? Do I need to take all the prenatal tests? Questions about exercise, nutrition, drugs during labor, and even finances can usually be answered by your trusted health-care worker whether he or she is a general practitioner, obstetrician or midwife.

Thom and I researched our options, prayed about them and decided to have all natural deliveries in a hospital setting. Then we had to find a doctor. After going to three different obstetricians that did not seem very open to natural childbirth, a friend called recommending her doctor. "He's nice," she said.

I went to see him and found out he does not perform abortions, is open to natural childbirth and practices alone, so I would only have one doctor. The quality that attracted me the most to my doctor, however, is his kindness. Just as my friend told me, he is nice. I'm never afraid to ask questions and I'm not intimidated by him. He's open, easy to talk to and caring while also maintaining a professional posture.

Choosing the right doctor is an important step in pregnancy. Your life and your baby's life are entrusted to his or her hands. If you don't have a doctor or you're dissatisfied, ask the Lord's guidance in helping you find the right one.

Prayer starter: Father, I know You care about all the decisions I have to make. Thank You for helping me find the right doctor to deliver this child. Give him or her wisdom and discernment concerning me and my baby.

DAY 80

"He who finds a wife finds what is good and receives favor from the Lord" *(Prov. 18:22).*

Lately I've been getting teary-eyed at the drop of a hat. Hearing a dog whine, "The Star-Spangled Banner," the laughter of my children—these things don't normally make me want to cry. But I'm not normal; I'm pregnant. Watching the babies on the diaper commercial on TV makes me think of the one I'm carrying now. I get so excited and happy, I cry!

Now that we've gone through this a few times, Thom understands. He doesn't complain about my quirks. He seems to enjoy helping me as my changing body affects my brain and emotions.

When you need a few more hugs and kisses—when your entire being cries out for a banana split at midnight—when you want to weep at the TV commercials for long-distance telephone service—remind your husband that when he found you, he found a good thing, and that as a result of marrying you, *he* finds favor with the Lord. What a nice verse. It makes me feel better already.

Prayer starter: Lord, thank You for the institution of marriage. Thank You for my husband. Help us during this special time in our relationship to prepare for parenthood together. Help us to draw closer to You and closer to each other.

DAY
81

"Can a mother forget the baby at her breast and have no compassion on the child she has borne? Though she may forget, I will not forget you" *(Is. 49:15).*

Think about your own birth. Did you come into the world wanted and loved by your parents? Or were you viewed as an accident, a mistake?

Rejection for some people started in the womb. Unchecked, feelings of rejection can spawn any number of emotional problems from bitterness to resentment to hate. The good news for those who have been rejected is that through Jesus Christ we have forgiveness of sins. We who have been forgiven must also forgive. As we forgive all of those who hurt us, the wounds begin to heal.

We can't return to the womb and try all over again to enter a world devoid of hurts and rejection. But we can be born again by God's Spirit, given a clean slate, made into a new creation. Ask God to examine your life. He'll show you where you need forgiveness and whom you need to forgive.

It's hard to imagine, but even a mother can forget her child. But God loves us always, never leaving nor forsaking us. As expectant mothers, now is a good time to clean house, to examine our lives and allow God to do His work in us. Our babies deserve mothers who are emotionally whole!

Prayer starter: Lord, I invite You to look deep within my heart and show me any wickedness. Forgive me, Father, when I get off Your path. Help me to uproot the problems in my life. Empower me by Your Spirit to forgive those who have hurt me. I pray for this baby that she'll not experience rejection from me in any way. If I have any attitude whatsoever that could be remotely received by my baby as rejection, show it to me, so that I can repent and shower my baby with love and acceptance.

DAY

82

"Blessed is the man who fears the Lord, who finds great delight in his commands. His children will be mighty in the land; the generation of the upright will be blessed" *(Ps. 112:1-2)*.

One Sunday when I was pregnant with Benjamin, Thom and I along with Holly and David went to sing and minister in a church.

On the way, we sang and prayed for the service and generally had a joyful ride through the country. We arrived early, before the doors to the church were open, so we bought some orange juice and muffins and sat in the car outside the church eating, drinking and reading our Bibles. Psalm 112:1-2 seemed to jump off the page at me. Right away I thought maybe God was giving me a special nugget from His Word that would apply especially to my unborn child.

"Holly, David, are you strong and mighty? Let me feel your muscles," I said. They flexed for me. "God's making you strong because Daddy and I love and serve Him. Listen to this verse from Psalms." I read them the verse while they continued trying to make muscles, giggling at each other.

I prayed and claimed this verse throughout my pregnancy with Benjamin. He certainly is a strong little boy physically, but I think God will also bless him and all of our children with spiritual strength.

Prayer starter: Lord, I love You and want to serve You. I take You at Your Word and believe that the child I'm carrying will indeed be mighty. I believe You're blessing this generation of children.

DAY

83

"Now, my son, the Lord be with you, and may you have success....Be strong and courageous. Do not be afraid or discouraged" *(1 Chron. 22:11,13)*.

When King David prepared to leave his throne, he gave advice to his successor, Solomon, his son. "May the Lord give you discretion and understanding," he said. "You will have success if you are careful to observe the decrees and laws that the Lord gave Moses for Israel."

Some might call David, who committed adultery and had a man murdered, a hypocrite for instructing his son to obey the Lord. Often in the Psalms, David cries out to God in fear and discouragement. Yet to Solomon he says, "Don't be afraid or discouraged."

If we in the modern world can see David's sins, his repentance and his restoration to God, surely Solomon knew his father's heart.

David wasn't a hypocrite for instructing Solomon to do things he could not accomplish himself. He was being real, open and honest. He wanted Solomon to succeed, so he gave him good advice.

What an encouragement to a son or daughter! Our children will find trouble in this world, but if we're honest with them and let them see our faults and shortcomings, then we can also show them how God helps us overcome our weaknesses. David was a role model for repentance and restoration to God. We should be, too.

Prayer starter: Lord, forgive me when I fall short of Your best for me. Help me to be a good role model for my child, doing the best I can to live a godly life. When I fail You or my child, help me to be honest and to confess my faults, so that my child, too, will know how to find restoration in You.

DAY 84

"May the Lord make you increase, both you and your children. May you be blessed by the Lord, the Maker of heaven and earth" *(Ps. 115:14-15).*

I'm crying again. I just called a friend who moved out of town a few years ago after having her seventh baby. She gave me a pattern for maternity slacks which I never returned, and I wanted to let her know I just found it in my maternity clothes.

Her daughter answered the phone and told me her mother was eight months pregnant with baby number eight! So why am I crying? I don't know. I'm happy for my friend. I admire her greatly. She loves God, she's smart, and she has a great husband, meaningful work and seven beautiful, well-behaved children. She's blessed!

Although we haven't spoken to one another for months, I feel a warm, sisterly bond.

Prayer starter: Lord, Maker of heaven and earth, once again I thank You for the child You're forming within me. I pray You'll bless this child! Bless my friend and her baby. Pour out Your love on all the expectant mothers right now. Nurture the love we have for each other; help us to encourage one another and point our children to You.

DAY 85

"And God said, "Let the land produce living creatures according to their kinds" *(Gen. 1:24).*

In the natural world, animals reproduce their own kind. Cows bear cows. Lions bear lions. Although I've had dreams that my baby was a hot dog or a frog, the baby will be human. (When people ask Thom if he wants a boy or girl, he tells them, "Considering I'm the dad, we're just praying it's a human being.") Yes, all joking aside, humans produce humans.

In the soul and spiritual worlds, the same principle is true. Psalm 7:14 says, "He who is pregnant with evil and conceives trouble gives birth to disillusionment." If you're a troublemaker, you'll get yourself in trouble.

If, however, you sow goodness and kindness, love, mercy, justice, forgiveness and joy in others, these qualities will grow in you.

Prayer starter: Lord, remind me that I reap what I sow. Just as this tiny baby was conceived in love and will grow to be a child, a fruit of my husband's and my love, so let Your Spirit planted within me bear fruit for Your kingdom.

DAY 86

"They [the older women] can train the younger women to love their husbands and their children" *(Titus 2:4).*

One of my friends, who is eight months pregnant, called me with an offer I couldn't refuse. If I'd go shopping and serve as a consultant to her for items she needed for the baby, she'd buy dinner. We went to a local mall and had a nice time, scrutinizing every store that had a baby department. She was amazed at the wide variety of choices available for all sorts of items. I told her about all the different types of bottles I tried and which seemed to work the best. We talked about the choices in breast pumps, T-shirts and styles of bibs. She bought an infant car seat which was light and small enough to carry into a restaurant and fit onto a chair, yet sturdy enough to last through a couple of babies.

I was happy that after three babies I had learned something to share with my friend. The very best lesson I've learned about being a mom, however, has nothing to do with choosing the right brand of diapers or when the right time is to start your child on solid food. The greatest lesson is that I've learned to love in a way I never thought was possible.

It's not my nature to put others first, to sacrifice my own needs and wants for someone else's. I know I should, but I never seemed to be able to do this, even with Thom. Yet I tend to the needs of my children automatically—feeding, clothing, bathing, playing with them and just *loving* them.

Love your children. Let them know you love them. If we mothers really learn this lesson, our children's generation will have a solid, secure foundation upon which to build their lives.

Prayer starter: Father, teach me to love with Your kind of love. Help me to love my children. Help me to encourage other women to love their children and their husbands. I pray that my baby and the babies of other expectant mothers will be born strong and secure, surrounded by love.

DAY
87
"Keep your lives free from the love of money and be content with what you have" *(Heb. 13:5).*

The first baby gift I ever received was a Calvin Klein bib which I received when I was about three months pregnant with Holly. Thom and I were sponsoring Amy Grant in concert in Pittsburgh. After hearing I was pregnant, the promoter of the concert tour visited one of Pittsburgh's exclusive stores, bought the bib and gave it to me the night of the concert.

It really is a nice bib, made of blue denim backed by red terry cloth. I've used it for all the children, and I remember that concert promoter fondly when Benjamin slops spaghetti all over his hand-me-down designer bib. It probably cost more than most of the outfits the children wear.

I suppose it would be nice to clothe my children in the finest apparel and have them sleep in the best cribs that money can buy. But brand-name cribs and designer bibs are not very high on my priority list. We belong to a church that has many young families. Baby clothes and cribs are traded around, so that no one really *needs* to spend a fortune on items for the baby.

Prayer starter: Lord, help me to be content with what I have and not covet money and the things money buys. Thank You for Your provision for me and my family. Help this baby to have an abundance of love and a heart to serve You.

DAY 88

"Do not let your hearts be troubled. Trust in God" *(John 14:1).*

Driving home from a concert late at night, an opossum ran in front of the car. Thom slowed down, while the opossum, frozen with fear, stared at the headlight momentarily, then scurried into the woods.

"Did you know, children, that opossums are like kangaroos? They carry their babies in pouches," Thom said. "Animals with pouches are called *marsupials*," Mr. Science adds.

"I didn't know that," I said, pondering the possibilities of being an opossum. "It must be nice for the opossum mom to take a peek into her pouch to make sure her baby's OK. I wouldn't mind being able to do that right now."

No sooner had I said it than I felt the conviction of the Lord. "Trust Me, My daughter. I've got everything under control."

It's better that I can't actually see my baby while she develops. I must trust and believe that God is forming this child perfectly, according to His plan.

Prayer starter: Lord, forgive me when I take my eyes off of You. Help me be continually reminded that You are in control of my life and the life of this unborn child. I trust in You, so I am not troubled.

DAY
89 "Make a joyful noise unto the Lord" *(Ps. 100:1, KJV).*

Thom had concern in his voice as he talked to our friend John on the telephone. After he hung up he said, "John's coming over to talk. He's going through a real trial and he needs some help and support."

"Remember, you said you'd watch the children while I run some errands. Can you talk to John and watch three kids?" I asked.

"Sure, no problem."

I left the house and shot up a few quick prayers for John. After quickly doing my errands, I returned to the house and heard very joyful noises pouring out from my basement. Thom and John were playing guitars while David beat on the drums, Holly played the harmonica, and Benjamin danced.

"Let me take the kids now so you two can talk," I offered.

"I don't want to talk now. We're having too much fun," John said. There's nothing like praising the Lord with a joyful noise to take your mind off yourself and the trials and tribulations of life. The problems will have to be faced, but with God in the midst of them, you know you'll have the power you need to overcome.

Prayer starter: Lord, help me to make a joyful noise to You in all kinds of circumstances, even when I'm feeling down. I pray that this baby will likewise learn to praise You. When the trials and problems of life come, help me to teach my children by example to praise You.

How do you feel? How much weight have you gained? Have you told family and friends your good news? Is God blessing the fruit of His peace in your life? Have you had the chance to pray with your husband about your baby and this pregnancy?

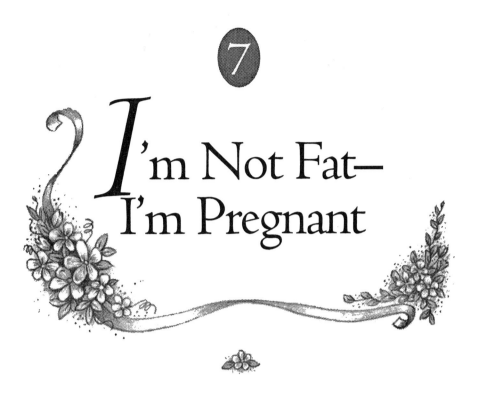

I'm Not Fat— I'm Pregnant

D A Y S   9 0 – 1 1 9

MONTH FOUR The baby's growing fast! By the end of the month he or she will weigh about six ounces and measure around eight inches. Facial and head features become more defined, and the eyes, nose, mouth and ears are completed. The baby's muscles are able to contract, and slow eye movements begin. Some say that as early as the twenty-sixth week the baby can hear the mother's voice. It is possible this month that you will have a fluttery, bubbly feeling that is actually the baby moving! This "quickening" occurs at different times for each individual. With my first baby I didn't feel movement until the sixth month. With the next two I felt it much earlier. If you have any fears or concerns about not feeling movement, tell your doctor. The sound of a strong steady heartbeat can be reassuring that all is well.

Prayer starter: Father, I know Your hand of blessing is constantly on this growing baby. I pray the first sounds this baby hears will be joyful and life-giving.

DAY 90

"Bless the Lord, O my soul, and all that is within me, bless his holy name" *(Ps. 103:1, KJV).*

I'm trying to get ready for a party where I'll see old friends and relatives for the first time in years. I'm too small for maternity clothes and too big for everything else. What I need is a T-shirt like one I saw on a woman in the doctor's office that read, "I'm not fat—I'm pregnant!" That's really what my vain self wants to declare to the world and what I'll surely tell Lori who looks thin and lovely, even when she's nine months pregnant. I've settled on a waistless blue dress that my sister made during her first pregnancy. Despite the fact that I feel rather unattractive in my hand-me-down outfit, I'm suddenly filled with awe and excitement for the miracle growing inside of me. With hands on my expanding belly, I wonder about this little one, this child who is causing my figure to grow rounder by the day. Gazing in the mirror at the chubby woman in a blue maternity dress, the reality hits. I'm pregnant!!! I'm really going to have a baby!

"Bless the Lord, O my soul, and all that is within me, bless His holy name."

Prayer starter: Lord, I'm filled with praise and thanks to You for Your gift of life. May all that is within me, even this little one, bless Your holy name!

DAY 91

"The fruit of the Spirit is...gentleness" *(Gal. 5:22).*

I'll never forget how delicate and beautiful Holly looked to me as a newborn. Coming home from the hospital at six pounds ten ounces, she fit neatly into one of Thom's big hands. Be gentle—be gentle, I kept telling myself, somehow afraid she could break. Later, when Holly had just turned two, David was born. Taking Holly's pudgy little hand and stroking David's head with it, I told her, "Be gentle—be gentle."

Just as we adults know how to be physically gentle with our

children, God treats His children gently in the spiritual realm. Isaiah 40:11 says God "gently leads those that have young." He's especially sensitive and gentle to us expectant mothers.

He's gentle in His discipline. When the Pharisees threatened to stone the woman caught in adultery, Jesus intervened with the fruit of gentleness. "Go now and leave your life of sin," He says in John 8:11. He did not judge harshly, embarrassing and condemning the woman. He dealt with her gently, not because He was a weak man, but because He had the spiritual strength to discern her heart, her needs.

We mothers need to develop gentleness in our spirits to parent our children properly. Gentleness is often translated "meekness," which in our modern language is often used to describe a quiet or weak person. Such is not the case! Christ, the King of kings, could be gentle because of His authority and great strength. As parents we can also be gentle, because we are the authority to our kids. Our goal, like the Lord's, is to nurture fruit in our children. Therefore we ought to emulate His gentleness to us in raising our own children.

Prayer starter: Lord, I pray that You'll bless me with the fruit of gentleness. Teach me Your gentle ways. I pray that this fruit will be abundant in my life as I raise my child so that he, too, will bear the fruit of gentleness in his heart and actions.

DAY 92

"For he will command his angels concerning you to guard you in all your ways; they will lift you up in their hands, so that you will not strike your foot against a stone" *(Ps. 91:11-12).*

Thom was mowing the grass; the children were inside coloring. The phone rang, and Holly answered. She called to her father who left the mower running and dashed inside to answer the telephone. Thom did not notice little David go outside, until with horror he saw David put his foot curiously under the swirling blades.

Thom dropped the receiver and ran to David who was screaming in pain. He scooped the child into his arms and rushed into the house, praying as he ran, "Help me, Jesus!"

The top of David's tennis shoe was sheared by the mower blade.

Thom gingerly removed the shoe and bloody sock and saw, to his surprise, a very superficial cut on the top of one toe.

Thom bandaged the toe, thanking God there had been no major injury. He had a serious discussion with David about never touching a lawn mower.

For Thom's birthday, I bought a glass serving dish, placed the sheared tennis shoe in it, with the verse "He shall give his angels charge over thee" to serve as a reminder to pray that angels would be sent to protect our family.

Prayer starter: Lord, thank You for Your protection. Thank You for caring enough for us that You will send angels to help us. Please protect this baby from any harm.

DAY
93
"He that hath two coats, let him impart to him that hath none" *(Luke 3:11, KJV).*

Krista gave me a white and brown maternity dress today. I recognized it as one that I'd seen Becky wear. When I wore the dress to church, Janet came up to me and said, "You look great in my dress."

As I grow larger and larger, I know the women in my church will pass on more clothes. Some people don't like clothes swapping. But I think it's a great idea. Not only does it help me have outfits to wear, but it binds me closer to my sisters in Christ. The maternity clothes exchange is just another example of how God's economy works, how He indeed provides for all of my needs.

Prayer starter: Lord, thank You for taking care of my needs through Your riches in glory. Thank You for loving friends and sisters in Christ. I pray You'll teach me how to be a friend and show me how I can be a blessing to others, just as others have blessed me.

DAY 94

"Since we have these promises, dear friends, let us purify ourselves from everything that contaminates body and spirit, perfecting holiness out of reverence for God" *(2 Cor. 7:1).*

A well-balanced diet does not mean McDonald's for breakfast, Wendy's for lunch and Pizza Hut for dinner. I have to remind myself that the baby relies on me for nourishment. If I contaminate myself with fatty fast foods laden with chemicals and preservatives, I jeopardize my little one's health as well as my own.

I also need to feed my spirit with God's Word and avoid contamination from the ungodly sights and sounds around me. This may mean turning off the television and radio. I can't do much about the pollution in the air, but I can be careful not to add to the pollution in my mind and heart if I monitor the input I receive and say no to evil thoughts.

Prayer starter: Help me, Lord, to eat nutritious, well-balanced meals that will provide strength, energy and health to me and my developing child. Bless the food and drink I consume and guard my system from contamination. Give me Your wisdom and discernment to avoid contaminating my thoughts and actions.

DAY 95

"My sheep listen to my voice; I know them, and they follow me" *(John 10:27).*

Thom and I were singing for teenagers at a community center. After sharing our testimonies and encouraging the kids to seek God's will for their lives, a young girl came up to me with questions. ''How can I know what God wants me to do? I have to make all kinds of decisions about college—where to live, what to study. I want to hear from God, but I hear so many different suggestions and get conflicting advice. What should I do?''

God speaks to us through His Word. If I stray from daily Bible reading, I may not notice it immediately, but I do get more confused about my priorities. But when I communicate continually with God

in prayer and praise and through reading His Word, I'm rarely un-
sure of what I'm supposed to be doing.

"Are you praying about it and reading your Bible every day?"
I asked her.

"Well, I've prayed, but I hardly ever read my Bible."

"Start reading every day," I told her. "You'll start recognizing
what is God's voice and what is not."

*Prayer starter: Father, help me daily to seek Your face, read Your
Word and recognize Your will for my life. You know I need guidance
and direction on being a mother. Help me. I want Your best for my
child.*

DAY 96

**"Consider how the lilies grow. They do not labor or spin...If
that is how God clothes the grass of the field, which is here
today, and tomorrow is thrown into the fire, how much more
will he clothe you"** *(Luke 12:27-28).*

Thom and I thought we were singing for a Sunday evening church
service for adults. I wore a green maternity dress and black pumps.
I felt a little frumpy-looking and looked much more than three months
pregnant. But normal clothes didn't fit!

To my horror, when we arrived at the church, it turned out to be
a youth rally with teens from five or six churches. Everyone, including
the pastors and adults, was wearing jeans. I felt like a jerk but figured
there was nothing I could do but go ahead and try to act cool, even
though I felt as if I looked very uncool.

I mentioned to one of the sponsors that I felt uncomfortable in my
dress and old lady shoes. To my surprise, this woman I'd never met
invited me to run quickly to her house and find something different
to wear. Between her and her teenage daughters, she thought I'd fit
into something.

In minutes I had an outfit: black jeans, a big bulky sweater and
even a different pair of shoes. Back at the youth rally, I blended right
in and actually felt good about myself. The crowning touch happened
when a ninth-grade boy, mistaking me for one of the teens, tried
to get friendly. (OK, the lights were dim.) When I told him I was

thirty-something and pregnant with my fourth child, he was pretty surprised.

I don't know if my appearance changed the way the kids received our message. But I do know I was able to communicate more effectively, not thinking I looked like a geek.

Prayer starter: Father, thank You for Your provision. I'm sorry that I ever worry or fret, because I know You care about me and my needs, and You are able to supply me even with clothes I can wear at this time. Help me adjust to the fact that my body is changing and know in my heart that it's all for a good reason!

DAY
97 "I am the Lord that healeth thee" *(Ex. 15:26, KJV).*

I feel pretty good this morning. Praise God. Come to think of it, I felt good yesterday and the day before that. Could it be that the morning sickness is gone and that I'm going to feel great until the delivery of this child? I hope so.

I can't believe I've felt good for a few days, and I'm just now acknowledging it and thanking God.

Prayer starter: Father, thank You for my health and strength. Thank You for daily blessing and strengthening my baby as he grows in my womb.

DAY
98 "But as many as received him, to them gave he power to become the sons of God" *(John 1:12, KJV).*

I heard the sermon title, "But as many as received him, to them gave he power...." I ended the sentence in a variety of ways, knowing that I have received Jesus Christ. I have the power to become a nurse who cleans cuts, kisses hurts and removes splinters; a seamstress who repairs rips, fixes zippers, shortens and lengthens dresses and slacks; a dietitian and chef who designs delicious, nutritious meals and serves them in an attractive, appetizing fashion; a laundress who can remove pizza sauce stains even after they've been covered with chocolate and sealed with peanut butter; a spiritual genius who can explain and pray for a child who's crying because "the big kids won't let me play."

Yes, God has given me not only the power to become His child, but He's given me the power to become a mother. I hadn't touched a sewing machine since junior high school and I *never* tried to comfort a child who was too little for the neighborhood ball game. I didn't even know I would need these skills, yet God gave me the power to become the mom I need to be.

I know He'll give me the power by His Spirit to rejoice in Him the next several months as I carry this baby. He'll give the power I'll need on delivery day.

Prayer starter: Lord, conform me to Your image. Help me be the mother I should be to the child You're forming inside me. Give me wisdom, insight and discernment to raise this child for Your glory. I thank You that through Your power I can become a mother whose children will serve You with joy.

DAY 99

"The blueness of a wound cleanseth away evil: so do stripes the inward parts of the body" *(Prov. 20:30, KJV).*

This verse makes me think of stretch marks—who wants them? Surely not I. Some doctors say these "stripes of motherhood" are inevitable. Others say that at least ninety percent of pregnant women get these tiny to large bluish-red marks as the skin stretches to accommodate the growing child.

If you're like me, you may invest in creams to rub into your skin to try to avoid earning your "stripes." These products can't hurt you and probably feel good. But those who escape stretch marks do it with or without the creams and lotions. Good, elastic skin tone, either inherited or nurtured through years of proper diet, and drinking plenty of water are the current explanation for women who escape stretch marks. So drink your water and eat right before your belly gets too big! I had two babies with absolutely no stretch marks and without paying much attention to rubbing my belly with oils. Then with Benjamin I earned my stripes. They've faded to slender silver lines, but I somehow feel it's inevitable that they'll expand as I do this time around.

Solomon wasn't talking about stretch marks when he wrote about stripes on the belly, however. Looking at this verse in the Amplified Bible sheds more light on its meaning: "Blows that wound cleanse away evil, and strokes [for correction] reach to the innermost parts." Sometimes correction and discipline seem to hurt us, but godly correction will reach us deep inside.

Prayer starter: Lord, I place my life and the life of this baby into Your hands again today. Show me by Your Spirit how to live day by day. Correct me where I need correction, because I want my thoughts and actions always to be in Your perfect will.

DAY 100

"I have never seen the righteous forsaken or their children begging bread. They are always generous and lend freely; their children will be blessed" *(Ps. 37:25-26).*

My friend Chris told me that when she discovered she was pregnant with her fourth child she panicked. Her husband had lost his job, and she feared the family would not be able to make ends meet.

"How will we feed this baby, Lord?" she cried.

God assured her that He would not forsake her and that her children would not have to beg for bread. He prompted her to read Psalm 37:25. When she looked up the verse, she saw it was followed by the statement that the righteous are generous and their children blessed. She said she began to confess this verse to herself and her unborn baby. She gave freely what she had.

Her family endured the tough time, and just as God promised, the baby was born blessed, never going hungry. Her husband, out of work for a year, found a good job and can now care for his family and continue in the generosity that characterizes the sincere Christian.

Prayer starter: Lord, thank You for reminding me that You provide for all of my needs. I give You again all the financial needs that will be required to raise this child, knowing that You will provide and bless my child.

DAY 101

"Do not be terrified; do not be discouraged, for the Lord your God will be with you wherever you go" *(Josh. 1:9).*

My doctor thought I looked a little larger than I should, so he advised me to have an ultrasound examination. After doing so, I discovered both the good news that my baby is fine and the bad news that a fist-sized fibroid tumor is growing in my uterine wall.

My doctor explained that these are fairly common and that, while it was possible the tumor could grow and pose a threat to me or my child, this was highly unlikely. Knowing I prefer totally natural deliveries, he cautioned me that I should mentally prepare for the possibility of a cesarean section.

I heard what he had to say, but I can't open my mind enough to entertain the possibility of having the baby removed surgically from my belly. I know if a doctor told me I would die or my baby would be harmed if I don't agree to a cesarean, I would go through with it. But at this stage in my pregnancy I have the faith to believe my problem will go away or won't pose a threat on labor day.

If you have a complication or problem, I'd recommend getting a second opinion. Pray and ask God either to remove the complication or give you the wisdom to deal with it and overcome.

Prayer starter: Lord, I know that You are with me now and that You'll be with me until my day of delivery, going through the entire process. I need not be afraid, because You are my strength and my shield.

DAY 102

"But Jesus said, Suffer little children, and forbid them not, to come unto me: for of such is the kingdom of heaven" *(Matt. 19:14, KJV).*

One of my friends, hearing that I was surprised with this pregnancy, told me that his conception had been an accident. "My mother said she almost called me 'Oops!' instead of Joe."

Laughing, he added, "She told me I was the best mistake she ever made."

"When did you hear all this? Do you remember?" I asked him.

"Yes, I guess I was about thirteen or fourteen. At the time it really bothered me—I have two older brothers, and I figured that she loved them more than she loved me. But the Lord really helped me get over that. I know He loves me, and I know my mom and dad do, too."

I don't know if Joe's mother was right or wrong in telling him he was "the best mistake she ever made." But I do know that the love of God covers a multitude of the mistakes we parents make. By leading our children to a personal relationship with Jesus Christ, we introduce them to the Answer to all of their problems.

Prayer starter: Lord, give me wisdom to be the mother You want me to be. Give me a sense of humor, along with that wisdom, as my child goes through the ups and downs of life. Help me set a good example of a person whose life is greatly enriched and strengthened through a personal relationship with Christ. Help my child's heart to have a longing to "come unto You."

DAY 103

"Praying always...that utterance may be given unto me, that I may open my mouth boldly" *(Eph. 6:18,19, KJV).*

One of my pregnant friends works in an atmosphere that is always filled with smoke. Knowing that tobacco smoke not only contaminates the smoker and other persons in the vicinity who must breathe the smoke, but it also affects the unborn child, my friend decided she may have to quit work. She had intended to work as long as possible; she and her husband planned their budget around her working at least seven months.

My suggestion to her, rather than to quit her job over the situation, was to talk to her co-workers. Confrontation is hard, but I predicted people would understand her concerns for her unborn child.

"Pray about it. Ask God to give you the right words to say, then ask to meet with your colleagues. Tell them how you feel and explain that you're willing to quit your position if they can't stop smoking in the room where you work. But make it clear that you will not jeopardize the health of your baby by inhaling their smoke.''

Guess what? She did it. Her friends at work not only were understanding and set up a ''smoking area'' in the office, but one even praised her honest attitude and concern for her baby.

Prayer starter: Lord, help me to do what I need to do to protect the health and welfare of my baby. Empower me by Your Spirit to have the boldness to speak to others when I know I must.

DAY 104

"My son, hear the instruction of thy father, and forsake not the law of thy mother: for they shall be an ornament of grace unto thy head and chains about thy neck" *(Prov. 1:8-9, KJV).*

What does this proverb say to me?
1. A child should heed instruction from his father and mother. Therefore:
    a. The mother and father must be united in philosophy, doctrine and teachings or the child will hear conflicting voices. Parents must be consistent in their instruction.
    b. Both the father and the mother have responsibilities to nurture, train and discipline the children.
2. The mother and father must both be open vessels, willing to learn, hear from God and receive discipline if they're to instruct their children.
3. The godly teaching a child receives from his parents will equip him or her to take dominion over the earth. ''The ornaments of grace'' on their heads and ''chains about thy neck'' suggest the kind of royalty that ''King's kids'' need to do the work of the King of kings.

Prayer starter: Father, help my husband and me to pray for this child and discuss our parenting roles together, so that we may receive Your instruction and teaching for her. I pray this baby's head will be an ornament of grace and that she will walk with You as one of Your children.

DAY 105

"Speaking to yourselves in psalms and hymns and spiritual songs, singing and making melody in your heart to the Lord" *(Eph. 5:19).*

One of my children's playmates, Laura, who's three, was swinging on a swing set in a beautiful park. With sunlight streaming through the trees and the happy sounds of children playing, Laura began to sing one of her favorite songs: "He's a big guy, bigger than the swing set, bigger than the trees, bigger than that red house, bigger than the clouds...He's a big, big, big, big, big, big, wonderful guy."

"What's your daughter singing about?" I asked my friend, Laura's mother.

"Oh, she just makes up words to songs all the time. She thinks the song 'He's a Big God' is 'He's a Big Guy.' I don't correct her; I think the Lord is blessed to know that Laura understands He is bigger than everything—even bigger than her dad—the biggest guy she knows!"

Prayer starter: Lord, help me to have the heart of a little child, pure before You, full of joy and thanksgiving. As this baby's heart is growing in strength every day, prepare it even now to make melody to You. Bless these little lips and voice as they form to be ready to sing Your praise.

DAY 106

"Be careful for nothing; but in every thing by prayer and supplication with thanksgiving let your requests be made known unto God" *(Eph. 4:6, KJV).*

Thom called me with a tone of excitement in his voice. He found a house he wants me to see. It's a big, old Victorian home, within walking distance to our office and for sale by the owner. The owner's about to be foreclosed upon and is willing to let it go for what she owes.

I fell in love with it. It has plenty of space and enough charm to earn a spread in *Better Homes and Gardens* (after *much* cleaning, painting and repairs).

The children love it, too. Holly checked to see if the refrigerator would fit in the kitchen. When she found out it would, she knew this was the house she'd been praying for.

"Yes, Mom, I think that's the right house for us," she told me.

We made an offer, and we're waiting to hear from the owner. There's so much to think about with a new baby coming! Will I be moving when I'm nine months pregnant? I hope so!

Prayer starter: Just as Your Word says, I'm trying to be anxious for nothing in regard to the needs of my family and this baby specifically. I thank and praise You for Your provision and care for us. In obedience to Your Word, I pray that You will grant us the requests of our hearts and specifically provide for the needs we'll have in bringing a baby into the world. Thank You, Lord.

DAY
107 "He who has ears, let him hear" *(Matt. 11:15).*

How many times have I held a little child's face in my hands, stared him or her right in the eyes and asked, "Did you hear me?" I wish at times I could do that to my husband, pastor, friends, neighbors and a few relatives, but such an action would insult an adult.

Jesus knew how to express the importance of His message to adults with love. "He who has ears, let him hear," He says over and over again. Of course we have ears, but God wants us to listen carefully and respond in our hearts to what His Spirit is saying. He wants us to be teachable and receptive to His Word and to act on what we hear.

With this point in mind, my husband wrote a song called "If You've Got Ears." The first verse goes like this: "If you've got ears, then listen to my song. If you've got hands, then clap along. If you've got feet, let the dancing begin. If you've got a mouth, then join right in." Our children love to clap, dance and sing along, which helps illustrate the idea that listening requires at least an inward and very often an outward response from the hearer. Do you hear me?

Prayer starter: Lord, give me ears to hear what You're saying and a heart to obey and follow Your Spirit's leading. I pray that You'll bless this baby as his ears grow and develop.

DAY
108
"In my Father's house are many rooms; if it were not so, I would have told you. I am going there to prepare a place for you" *(John 14:2).*

"I just don't have enough room in this house, Lord," I whined, stuffing a box of toys under the piano which consumes a quarter of the space in our little living room. "No closets, no shelves. Every nook and cranny is packed. Where will I put a baby?"

Even as the words came out of my mouth, I felt guilty. God had provided us with this house when I was pregnant with Holly. It was quite spacious for a family of three. People all over the world live in much smaller spaces.

The words to a song Thom had written based on Matthew 19:16 jumped into my head: "Don't lay up your treasures here on earth where moth and rust destroy."

"OK, Lord, I can be happy with what I have, knowing that I'm storing treasure in heaven, where Jesus has provided a room for me. I trust that You'll help me to throw away junk, reorganize my space and somewhere, somehow find room for this baby. I'll try not to worry about it anymore," I reluctantly prayed.

I know God provides for my needs and my baby's needs, whether those include a crib, a car seat, clothes or a room to sleep in.

Prayer starter: Lord, thank You for assuring me that You provide for me and my family. I trust You to take care of all of my needs. Thank You for reminding me that my treasure is stored in heaven, where Jesus has prepared a place for me and my whole family.

DAY 109

"Thou wilt keep him in perfect peace, whose mind is stayed on thee: because he trusteth in thee" *(Is. 26:3, KJV).*

My sister was crying when she called. "Does pregnancy affect your brain? My life the last couple of days has been like an 'I Love Lucy' rerun."

Her Lamaze instructor had advised her to put her wedding band on a chain around her neck since her hands were swollen. One day she inadvertently flushed the ring down the toilet. The chain had broken on a button or something—she doesn't know how she did it, except she saw the symbol of her love and commitment swirl down the drain.

Another day, she threw her dirty clothes and shoes into the washing machine. When she put the load into the dryer, to her horror she discovered her very nice, expensive camera had been washed. ("Yes, I heard a lot of clunking, but I thought it was the shoes!" she said.)

Fortunately, she's married to a kind, understanding man.

Some people do feel a little batty during pregnancy. Maybe it's hormones. Maybe it's a touch of fear and anxiety. But we can have the mind of Christ. God will keep us in His peace, if we keep our minds on Him.

Prayer starter: Lord, thank You for Your peace which passes my human understanding. I pray for my brain and thoughts that they'll be healthy and sane and not in any way confused. As my baby's brain develops, help it function perfectly as You planned.

DAY 110

"But I would not have you to be ignorant, brethren, concerning them which are asleep, that ye sorrow not, even as others which have no hope. For if we believe that Jesus died and rose again, even so them also which sleep in Jesus will God bring with him" *(1 Thess. 4:13-14, KJV).*

I was in my fourth month of a previous pregnancy when tragedy struck our family. Thom's brother, David, who lived with us, played drums in our band and had become Thom's sounding board and confidante, was killed in a head-on collision. God gave us the hope that David was with Him, and the grace to go on, but for weeks Thom and I and the rest of Thom's family openly expressed our grief in losing our dear brother. I had never seen my husband cry and now we both wept in each other's arms.

I often wondered if through my own grief the developing child within me would be affected. At that time, God seemed to pour out an abundance of love and healing for our hurts.

When our first son was born, we knew God wanted us to call him David and that he would bring more joy to our lives than we could ever imagine. In the years since all this occurred, our hurts have healed, and our David has grown into a very expressive little guy who can make us laugh at the drop of a hat.

We all go through different circumstances in our lives while we're pregnant. As much as I'd like the world to revolve around me and my needs at times, I must have the strength to deal with the ups and downs of life. If you're experiencing a painful situation, be comforted that God knows and understands what you're going through. He will not leave you or the child inside you. My David is a reminder that God protected us and carried us through the grief to joy!

Prayer starter: Lord, thank You for the assurance of salvation for those who are in Christ Jesus. Thank You for this baby that's forming within me. Whatever happens to me during this pregnancy, help me to look to You for courage and strength to deal with every circumstance.

DAY 111

"And as Jesus passed by, he saw a man which was blind from his birth. And his disciples asked him, saying, Master, who did sin, this man, or his parents, that he was born blind? Jesus answered, Neither hath this man sinned, nor his parents: but that the works of God should be made manifest in him" *(John 9:1-3, KJV).*

Some women feel especially guilty about the sins of their past, afraid that something they've done will harm their babies. In this passage

Jesus made it clear that neither the blind man nor his parents had sinned and caused the blindness.

The devil is the one who tries to kill and destroy. Jesus came to give life abundantly. If the devil is trying to kill, harm or destroy you or your child, you can cling to the hope that greater is He that is in you than he that is in the world. If calamity comes, just as with this blind man, what the devil meant for evil, God can use for good. He healed the blind man, and He can heal any hurt or wound that some past sin has left on you.

Prayer starter: Lord, thank You for Your grace and mercy. I know there is no condemnation for those who are in Christ Jesus. Thank You for forgiveness of sins. I pray for wholeness and perfect health for my child and pray that no stupid, sinful act I committed will result in harm to him.

DAY 112

"My voice shalt thou hear in the morning, O Lord; in the morning will I direct my prayer unto thee, and will look up" *(Ps. 5:3, KJV).*

This morning in prayer I envisioned little children peeking in at me, hearing my praise, listening to my prayer. I knew it was God showing me His desire for me to be an example of a godly mother. So often my schedule gets rearranged. We work different shifts, staying up late for one reason or another, and I start my morning hurriedly without the Lord.

When this happens, my day just isn't as blessed as it is when I spend time with the Lord as soon as my eyes open. I know I need to direct my prayer to the Lord in the morning before all the action of the day starts. This helps me order my day and serves as an example for my children.

Prayer starter: Lord, help me to remember my commitment to seek You in the morning. Help me be an example to my children of a woman who directs her prayers to You, my God to whom I look in all circumstances.

DAY
113

"Yet, O Lord, you are our Father. We are the clay, you are the potter; we are all the work of your hand" *(Is. 64:8).*

We took the children to see a display of colonial American craftsmen and women at work. Some were spinning flax into yarn, while others wove the yarn into blankets. There were glass blowers, quilters, blacksmiths and tanners. Of particular interest were the potters, who quickly demonstrated to the children how a lump of messy gray clay could be formed into a beautiful vase. After the vase, pot or dish is formed, it's placed into the oven. After it's baked, the potter polishes, buffs and perhaps puts it back into the oven. The potter has different procedures for completing the pot depending on its purpose. A pot for baking is finished differently from a delicate dish.

Our babies are formed by God's own hand. Human life is a result of God's design. Just as the potter molds the pot, God forms our babies into His image. They're not the only ones. God molds us, too. He knocks off the excess clay, buffs and polishes and then puts us in the refining fire. Sometimes we need to be fired a few times and polished again, so that we're strong and beautiful vessels that He can use for His purposes.

Prayer starter: Lord, I trust that You're molding this baby's physical body perfectly according to Your divine plan. Mold his mind and spirit also, as he is formed. I pray that You will likewise mold me into the person You want me to be. I yield my thoughts and actions to You, to be formed by Your Spirit, so that my life reflects the image of Jesus Christ to the world around me.

DAY
114

"A scroll of remembrance was written in his presence concerning those who feared the Lord and honored his name" *(Mal. 3:16).*

I'm so happy that I kept journals throughout my pregnancies. I often turn to the day Benjamin was born. Here's what I wrote: "I drove myself home from the office when I thought the baby might be on the way. Thom came home, we prayed, and off we went! (Thank You, Lord, for Cathy, the Christian nurse who reminded me when I arrived, 'I can do all things through Christ who strengthens me.') We got to the hospital at 4:45 p.m. Benjamin arrived at 5:15. No stitches! Praise the Lord, I didn't even throw up!

"Benjamin Joseph was named and dedicated to the Lord in the recovery room. As soon as we got up to my room, Pastor Dudley and Grandpa came and blessed little Benjamin with special prayer.

"Lord, as You bless this new little one, please fill Holly and David's hearts with love for their new brother."

I turn to this page of my journal over and over and pray, "Lord, I really enjoyed this delivery. Can we do a repeat?" (I don't get a clear answer on this request.)

Malachi says that God is keeping a journal, actually a "scroll of remembrance" concerning His children. I have been blessed, and I hope my children will be, in seeing the prayers and God's answers to those prayers. I encourage you to do the same. My journal entries are unorganized and messy. Grocery lists sit beside sermon notes and the innermost cries of my heart. But with a little trimming, I can read my notes and see God's hand on my life. It builds my faith.

Prayer starter: Thank You, Lord, for Your care and concern for me and my growing child. Help me to remember Your goodness; help me to have concrete examples to tell my children of how You lovingly hear and answer prayer.

DAY 115

"Let the beloved of the Lord rest secure in him, for he shields him all day long, and the one the Lord loves rests between his shoulders" *(Deut. 33:12).*

"Did you know that God gives piggyback rides?" my friend Katie asked me.

Knowing this was a baited question I replied, "No, please tell me about it."

Katie, who's expecting her eighth child, showed me this verse in Deuteronomy which portrays the Lord's protection. "How can a person rest between the Lord's shoulders? Only if God's giving a piggyback ride!'' Katie said.

Not only is God shown as protector, but Scripture paints a picture of the Lord as a loving playful dad who carries his kids on his back. I think of Thom who somehow manages to carry our three little ones all at once. I know it won't be long before another adoring pair of pudgy arms will reach up to him saying, ''Daddy, I want to ride on your back!''

Prayer starter: Lord, thank You for Your love and protection. Thank You for precious nuggets in Your Word that fill my mind with pictures of You that I can understand. I pray for Your protection for the baby I'm carrying; I pray that he will come to know You as a loving Father. Bless my husband as he prepares for parenthood. Mold him into Your image as a provider and protector and a loving, playful dad as well.

DAY 116

"I give thee charge in the sight of God, who quickeneth all things" *(1 Tim. 6:13, KJV).*

I was driving down a congested highway, one of the major arteries into the city of Pittsburgh, when I felt a fluttery feeling in my belly. I thought nothing of it. My friend Betsy and I were talking about the good times we'd had when we traveled together with our band. Betsy used to come along to watch children, pray with people, and take names and addresses of new converts in need of a Bible or church referral. In general, our conversation, as we drove through the traffic, testified to the good, fun things God had done in our lives.

Stopped at a red light outside one of my favorite gyro shops, I felt the flutters in my belly again. ''I have this funny feeling, Betsy, like butterflies in my stomach....'' No sooner had I said the words than I realized that my baby must be moving! I didn't get excited yet. I waited.

The next light was at a major intersection. I could see the jewelry store where Thom and I bought our wedding rings. There on the corner of West Liberty and Potomac Avenues, that baby moved again.

''Betsy! The baby's moving! I can feel it! I can feel it!''

I rejoiced at God's goodness. He had already ''quickened'' this child to move, but I couldn't help but be excited that now I could feel those movements.

Prayer starter: Thank You, Lord, for the life You've given me to nurture. Thank You that this baby is alive and kicking! I praise You, the Giver of life, for the miracle of children.

DAY 117

"When you open your hand, they are satisfied with good things" *(Ps. 104:28).*

Let me tell you about the miracle of the refrigerator that is too big to fit in our kitchen. When I was pregnant with Benjamin, our refrigerator broke on a day we were scheduled to sing at a church. We didn't have time to worry about the refrigerator; we had to get to our engagement.

I had a sense of peace that I didn't need to worry about the refrigerator, that God was taking care of everything supernaturally. I shared that feeling during the service, encouraging the congregation to walk one day at a time, relying on God for their every need. I told them about my broken refrigerator and the assurance God had given me about trusting Him to replace it. I remember saying, "I can't call Sears and ask them to deliver one, because I don't have money to pay for it. But I do know that God will work this situation out His way. It's in His hands."

The next day I received a call from a friend who runs a rescue mission in Pittsburgh. "Cathy, God told me to give you a refrigerator. When can I drop it off?"

"Right away!" I said, nearly falling off the chair.

A giant, side-by-side refrigerator was delivered. It didn't fit in my tiny kitchen, so it sits in the dining room taking up most of one wall.

I found out later that one of the mission's board members was in the congregation the night we sang. He heard our need and also knew that the mission had recently installed a refrigerated room to replace about ten refrigerators they had been using.

God is so good! Thom and Holly thought the refrigerator was too big. But they're not the ones who unpack the groceries, look for places to stack leftovers, and search for pickles and salad dressing. I love my refrigerator that doesn't fit in the kitchen and I thank God for it.

Prayer starter: Lord, thank You for Your provision for me and my family. I confess my fears again about the needs my family has regarding this new baby. I trust in You to provide for this baby and for the whole family.

DAY
118 "The Lord...will strengthen your frame" *(Is. 58:11b).*

My back started to hurt a few days ago. I haven't gained enough weight for the baby to be hurting my back, so I feared something might be wrong. After praying about it, I reread the section of *Husband Coached Childbirth* (Harper & Row) in which author Robert Bradley encourages expectant mothers to do "pelvic rock" exercises not eight times a day, as some pregnancy exercise books suggest, but 120 times, or forty times in a row, three times a day. The exercise is not difficult or strenuous. On all fours, you tuck in and flex both your abdomen and buttocks, putting your head down. When you relax, your head returns to an upright position with eyes straight ahead. I've done this exercise faithfully throughout all my pregnancies, and when it was time to push the baby out, I could feel these muscles I'd prepared at work. All three of my babies have been born with one or two pushing contractions.

Now I'm starting this exercise a little earlier than I have in previous pregnancies because my back is hurting. As I exercise I'll pray, using this promise from Isaiah.

Prayer starter: Lord, I believe that You strengthen my frame. I need that strength especially now that a child is growing within me. Show me what I can do to care for my body and keep it strong as it changes to accommodate my baby.

DAY
119

"Listen closely to my words...for they are life to those who find them and health to a man's whole body" *(Prov. 4:20b,22).*

I find myself wondering about people's life-styles when I'm in the grocery check-out line. The man behind me is holding a bag of chips, a liter of soda pop and two frozen dinners.

Probably a single guy.

The lady in front of me has money to splurge. She's buying gourmet cat food, steak fillets, real butter and a variety of deli items.

No one seems to care what I'm buying, but if they looked, they might be able to guess from my groceries that I'm pregnant or very strange (or maybe both). Tofu, pickles, peanut butter, pears, plain yogurt and a wide variety of grains, nuts and dried fruit fill my basket, along with frozen sweet treats, to satisfy my children and my cravings.

"Man does not live on bread alone but on every word that comes from the mouth of the Lord," the Bible says in Deuteronomy 8:3. If we want to be healthy and strong, we'll eat nutritious things, and we'll feed upon God's Word. A pregnant woman should not fast, because her growing baby needs certain nutrients daily that are not stored in the mother's body. Our spirits should likewise not fast. They should be fed daily from God's Word.

Prayer starter: Thank You, Lord, for the health and strength You give me. Thank You for building my physical body as You build my spirit. I pray the child I'm carrying will feed upon Your Word and be strengthened even as her physical body is strengthened.

How have you felt this month? What advice has your doctor given to you? How much weight have you gained? Have you been praying daily for your baby? What is your greatest concern at this time? Have you been praying for the fruit of gentleness to be manifested in your life? What has God shown you?

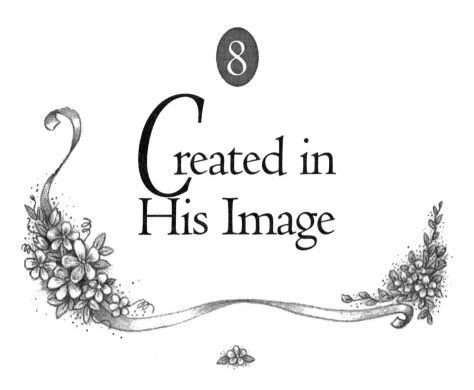

8

Created in His Image

D A Y S   1 2 0 – 1 4 9

MONTH FIVE   The baby continues to grow rapidly, weighing about a pound and measuring one foot by the end of the fifth month. Eyebrows and eyelashes appear, and hair grows on the head. Skeletal bones harden, muscles gain strength, and the heart beats louder and louder.

By now you probably look large enough for strangers to open doors and offer seats to you. Other mothers may nod in affirmative identification with you. Enjoy it! The whole world seems to smile on expectant mothers. And watch out, your navel could pop out at any time.

Prayer starter: Lord, I pray that, as this baby gains weight and strength, You will continue to bless and watch over the developmental process.

DAY
120

"So God created man in his own image, in the image of God he created him; male and female he created them" *(Gen. 1:27).*

"What does God look like?" my child asks.

Why doesn't someone write a book giving parents answers to our children's most-often-asked-and-nearly-impossible-to-answer questions. I suddenly realize that Someone has.

"The Bible says, honey, that God made you in His image. Do you know what that means? That means He made you to be like Him. We can't see God, so we don't know what He looks like. But the Bible says He is loving. He is patient. He is kind. He forgives. When you are loving and kind, patient and forgiving, you are acting in the special way that God wants you to. Did you know that?"

She nods at me slowly, then skips away to play. I'm sure the question will arise again, but right now my little girl is full of private thoughts to dwell upon.

Prayer starter: Father, I pray that the child inside of me will grow in Your image. I pray this baby will share Your love and kindness, peace and forgiveness, hope and patience with the world. Help me encourage the godly image that You've already placed inside this child.

DAY
121

"The fruit of the Spirit is...self-control" *(Gal. 5:22).*

With the fruit of self-control, we have the power to say no to fleshly passions that could harm us and our unborn children. This may involve total abstinence from obvious sins like sex outside of marriage and drug and alcohol abuse. It is hoped that such destructive behavior is non-existent in the expectant mother's life.

Self-control involves much more than controlling rage and conquering addictions. Self-control involves living a well-balanced life and exercising moderation.

Pregnancy provides a wonderful opportunity for us to examine our eating, drinking, exercise and sleep patterns. Caring for a new life within our own bodies gives added incentive to exercise self-control in our physical bodies.

Self-control is displayed differently by each individual, because we have unique weaknesses and varying tastes. I'm not tempted by a hot fudge sundae, but I must exercise self-control when faced with homemade bread, fresh from the oven, and real butter.

We must exercise self-control in our thoughts and emotions as well. I'm not prone to angry flair ups when people cross me. But I struggle with thoughts which, if turned into words, could be more destructive than a hasty punch in the nose.

We all want our children to develop good habits, to be able to exercise self-control in their lives. Drunkenness, drug addiction, fits of rage and gluttony are just some of the problems that occur in the out-of-control individual. We need to establish a pattern in our lives and in our children's lives to bear the fruit of godly self-control.

Prayer starter: Father, thank You for this opportunity to take a good look at myself and my habits. Forgive me for my lack of temperance. Show me the areas where I need work. I surrender control of my life to You. Teach me godly discipline so that I may live a self-controlled life. Bless this baby, and help me to sow seeds of temperance into his life, so that when he is older, those seeds will blossom into the fruit of self-control.

DAY
122 "Trust in God" *(John 14:1).*

I gained three pounds since my last visit to the doctor. Everything looks fine, he said. My doctor also said that now is the time to have an amniocentesis test if I want it. Amniocentesis is performed by inserting a long needle into the uterus through the abdomen wall and drawing out amniotic fluid. Through culturing and examining the fluid, birth defects such as Down's syndrome can be determined. The main purpose in diagnosing abnormalities in the baby at this stage is to give parents the option of abortion.

Since I would not abort my baby, I see no point in taking the risks in having the test done. About one in two hundred women experience infection or other complications that lead to miscarriage as a result of the procedure. This is much higher than the risk of Down's syndrome or other birth defects.

I don't turn down these tests because I'm against science or gaining knowledge. I pass on amniocentesis because I will not act on the information I receive, good or bad. I will trust in God.

Prayer starter: Lord, I put my trust in You to form this baby perfectly in Your image. I pray that You will guide me in the medical decisions I need to make regarding the healthy development and delivery of this child.

DAY
123
"So now I give him to the Lord. For his whole life he will be given over to the Lord" *(1 Sam. 1:28).*

How difficult it must have been for Hannah, after praying for years for a child, to give little Samuel, her firstborn, to the Lord. How could she leave him with the priests in the temple?

The Bible says she did it because she told the Lord she would. The Lord then used Samuel, who was set apart for His service even before conception, to be a prophet to his generation.

In my mind I know I can give my children to God, but I still cling to them as *precious* gifts. When this baby is born, and I dedicate him to the Lord in the recovery room of the hospital, I must remember Hannah. She kept her covenant with God by giving her Samuel willingly to Him. God greatly blessed both Hannah and Samuel; He used them.

I want God to use my children, too, as His instruments. I know this means giving them back to Him at birth, acknowledging that He knows what is best for them.

Prayer starter: Lord, this baby is dedicated to You. Help me as a mother to know how to raise this child in Your nurture and admonition, while releasing him into Your arms.

DAY
124
"Neither can you bear fruit unless you remain in me...I chose you to go and bear fruit—fruit that will last" *(John 15:4,16)*.

In intense labor with her second child, one of my friends said she called out to God, asking for help and strength. The Lord led her to the fifteenth chapter of John where Jesus spends much time talking about fruit. "I am the vine and you are the branches," He says. "If a man remain in me and I in him, he will bear much fruit; apart from me you can do nothing."

There in the labor room she examined her life and realized she needed to forgive a particular individual. After doing so in her heart, she came to a verse in the following chapter, John 16:21, where Jesus talks about a woman during labor. Knowing now that God was speaking to her, she read verse 23: "I tell you the truth, my Father will give you whatever you ask in my name...Ask and you will receive, and your joy will be complete."

She asked her husband to join her in prayer. She had the faith to believe God would take away the pain and hasten her labor. The doctor had told her he was ready to induce stronger contractions with drugs if her labor did not progress on its own. She had dilated only four centimeters after hours of hard contractions.

After prayer, my friend fell asleep. When the doctor came to examine her, he assumed her labor had stopped, since she was so relaxed. To his surprise, upon examination, the baby was crowning and ready for birth! She was rushed to the delivery room where her second daughter was born easily and quickly.

Prayer starter: Lord, I acknowledge that for me to produce fruit of any kind, whether it's a child of my own flesh and blood, a spiritual baby or the fruit of Your Spirit, I need You. I must remain in You, the vine. Prepare my heart even now to abide in You always, so that when I need You the most, I'll be able to hear Your voice and feel Your arms of love around me.

DAY

125 "I have learned to be content whatever the circumstances" (Phil. 4:11).

A letter arrived from the bank today denying our request for a mortgage to purchase the big house I was so sure the Lord wanted us to have. I called the bank.

"Surely there is something we can do. Can we reapply? Why were we turned down? Maybe there is a misunderstanding somewhere," I said with high hopes.

"There is nothing you can do. The matter is closed. A sheriff sale is scheduled, and I understand much higher bids which you cannot afford have been made. Forget it. Save your money and look for another house," he told me bluntly.

Thom was ministering with a team of American pastors and evangelists in Africa. I couldn't call him. I had no one to turn to, so I did what came naturally. I went to my bedroom and cried.

Holly came into my room, and I composed myself. She gave me a book to read and turned to the story she wanted to hear. "Contentment" was the name of it. (Honest!) The story told about a little girl who was upset because in school she was given a box of crayons that were old and broken, while the other children had nice new crayons to use. Recognizing her bad attitude right away, this saintly child asked for God's forgiveness then proceeded to draw the most beautiful picture, using the broken crayon tips to put wispy feathers on birds and the broad sides of the crayons with the paper ripped off to make bold dark strokes in the grass and sky. "Be happy with what you have" was the lesson.

I put Holly to bed and returned to my room where I began my repentance process. I gave all my desires and fears to the Lord in prayer again then flipped open my Bible. Here's where my eyes fell: "He tends his flock like a shepherd: He gathers the lambs in his arms and carries them close to his heart; he gently leads those that have young" (Is. 40:11).

The tears returned, only these were tears of healing and confirmation that God loved me in a special way because I am the pregnant mother of young children.

Prayer starter: Lord, thank You for Your reassuring Word that brings love and healing to me. Father, I am happy and content with what I have, and I thank You for all my material blessings. I trust You to provide all of my needs and all the needs this baby will have.

DAY 126

"Make level paths for your feet and take only ways that are firm. Do not swerve to the right or the left; keep your foot from evil" *(Prov. 4:26,27).*

Thom and I were driving with the children on an interstate highway. Thom mistakenly exited at the wrong place. Instead of getting right back on the highway, we had to go miles in the wrong direction, then retrace our steps back to the place the error was made, taking about an hour away from our progress.

Sometimes a little mistake is quite costly. The Bible cautions us to walk on firm, level paths. Jesus, the solid rock, provides a firm foundation for our walk through life. We should never choose a path that does not include Him. If we swerve, even slightly, to the left or right, we may get so far off course that it takes a long painful time to get back to our starting place.

Prayer starter: Father, I pray that Your Word would light my path, so that I can see where I should walk. Help me always to stay on course. I pray for my developing child that, while his bones are hardening and his feet are growing, You will bless them to walk in Your ways, never swerving to the right or left.

DAY 127

"Thou art worthy, O Lord, to receive glory and honour and power: for thou hast created all things, and for thy pleasure they are and were created" *(Rev. 4:11, KJV).*

During my first pregnancy Thom and I were scheduled to lead in worship at a weekend retreat with a group of people we did not know. On this retreat the first symptoms of what resulted in my miscarriage occurred. My doctor told me to stay in bed with my feet up.

I felt a little silly, holed up in bed while a group of strangers sang, prayed and received teaching.

But they weren't strangers for long. Through the walls of the retreat center, I heard the joyful singing: "Thou art worthy, thou art worthy...." I didn't know what was happening to my child or why I had to be in bed, but I felt the peace of God all around me. I found out later that others felt that peace, too.

Many of the women came to my room to pray and talk and to encourage me. One of them, Diane, brought a plaque the children had made in a craft class. It read, "Fear not, for I am with thee; be not dismayed for I am thy God who will comfort thee."

A week later I miscarried. The women who had prayed for me on the retreat sent cards and letters and stayed in touch. A bond had grown between us.

In no time at all I was pregnant again. I carried Holly to term, and she was born a beautiful, healthy baby. When the time came for this group's annual retreat, they asked us to sing again. We went with Holly, who was eleven weeks old.

Six years later, Diane, who had the children make the plaque for me, told me that those retreat experiences had deeply touched her heart. Shortly after the second retreat, she discovered she was pregnant with her first child. She became very ill but kept trusting in God, and her son was born, fine and strong. She told me just recently that in the recovery room she thought of me and that retreat and the worshipful song of the Lord that had been offered: "For thou hast created all things; and for thy pleasure they are and were created" (Rev. 4:11, KJV).

What a thrill it was to tell Diane, "I'm expecting my fourth child! I know that God has created your baby and mine for His pleasure. He is worthy!"

Prayer starter: Lord, thank You for creating me and the child that's in my womb right now. I do not understand the bad things that happen in my life, but I know that You do and You understand how I feel. You are worthy, Lord. I praise You and thank You for Your goodness.

DAY 128

"It was I who taught Ephraim to walk, taking them by the arms" *(Hos. 11:3).*

David revved with energy from his first few seconds out of the womb; at birth he wailed, kicked and squirmed. He grew quickly and could rock the sides of his bassinet at one month. He sat up and crawled early, so I wasn't surprised when he took his first step several months before the other children had. I remember Thom, the proud papa, egging him on, holding his hands at first so that he wouldn't stumble and fall.

Hosea paints a tender picture of our heavenly Father as he describes the Lord teaching Ephraim to walk. Ephraim here refers to the northern kingdom of Israel. If God cares enough to teach an entire nation to walk, how much easier it must be to teach me, one solitary woman?

Prayer starter: O Father, take me by the arms and teach me to walk! Help me to be the mother, the wife, the child You want me to be. Bless my husband, Lord. Help him to be a caring father who stretches out his arms to help this baby learn to walk and stretches out his heart and mind to nurture this baby in Your ways.

DAY 129

"With the help of the Lord I have brought forth a man" *(Gen. 4:1).*

Eve testified that it was with God's help that she bore Cain, her first son. Eve had messed up pretty badly just one chapter earlier, succumbing to the temptation of the devil and disobeying God. For her disobedience, she was cursed with the punishment that "in sorrow thou shalt bring forth children." Yet despite her sin and the curse, God was with her and helped her deliver Cain into the world.

We who have accepted Jesus Christ as our Savior have been set free from the curse. We are new creations, free from sin through the shed blood of Jesus Christ. If God helped Eve through labor and the delivery of Cain shortly after she erred so seriously, how much more will He be with us who have been reconciled to Him?

Prayer starter: Lord, thank You for Your redeeming power. I praise and thank You for providing a way through Jesus Christ for me to know You, to have fellowship with You. Help me throughout this pregnancy and at the time of delivery to deliver this baby safely and easily.

DAY 130

"If we are thrown into the blazing furnace, the God we serve is able to save us from it, and he will rescue us from your hand, O king. But even if he does not, we want you to know, O king, that we will not serve your gods or worship the image of gold you have set up" *(Dan. 3:17,18).*

King Nebuchadnezzar was pretty mad that Shadrach, Meshach and Abednego would not serve his gods, so he ordered that these three faithful Hebrews be burned to death. Even at the risk of undergoing such torture, the three Hebrews would not compromise nor deny their God. The furnace was heated seven times hotter than usual, and the soldiers who threw them into the blaze died from the heat. Shadrach, Meshach and Abednego had to go into the fire to demonstrate to the world that their God was willing and able to deliver them from harm. Had they died, they would have died serving God to the end. But they did not die—they were delivered miraculously—and King Nebuchadnezzar promoted them in the province of Babylon.

Sometimes God does not remove obstacles from our path, but He goes with us through the hard times, never leaving us and always loving us. As we journey the next few months, we may face some uncomfortable times. But let us look to the example of Shadrach, Meshach and Abednego, agreeing to serve God wholeheartedly and not our own selfish desires.

Prayer starter: Father, I vow to serve You, whether my road is rough or smooth. I pray for a safe, easy time of pregnancy and childbirth; but whether I feel great or not so good, I love You and will praise Your name.

DAY

131

"Finally, be strong in the Lord and in his mighty power. Put on the full armor of God so that you can take your stand against the devil's schemes" *(Eph. 6:10,11).*

If Jesus is Lord and Savior of your life, you've made a decision to be a child of God, to be reconciled to Him. That means you're on His side of a battle that began in antiquity and will last until the victorious return of Christ. Your identity as a child of God also makes you a target for the devil and his demons to harass. As a mother, you're an even greater foe to the devil because you have the opportunity to nurture and train another person for the Lord's service. If the devil can cripple and discourage you, he can probably get to your child as well.

"Put on the full armor of God," therefore, to defend yourself. This is an action you must take. Your unborn child can't make a conscious decision to battle the enemy, so you've got to put on the armor of God to protect the child within as well as yourself.

"Be strong in the Lord," Paul also tells the Ephesians. We need to tap into God's strength daily. Ask the Lord to fill you with His Spirit every morning when you pray.

During the next several days we're going to concentrate on the daily spiritual preparation that soldiers in God's army need to fight the fight.

Prayer starter: Father, I pray You'll give me the strength to do the work and fight the fight that's before me. Fill me anew with Your Spirit. I pray that Your divine protection will be upon this baby. Teach me how to put on the whole armor of God, so that I'll be equipped to do battle with the enemy.

DAY

132

"For we wrestle not against flesh and blood, but against principalities, against powers, against the rulers of the darkness of this world, against spiritual wickedness in high places" *(Eph. 6:12, KJV).*

Magazines and books bulge on bookstore and library shelves with information on childbirth, baby care, parenting and related subjects. It's good to be informed and to hear the advice child care experts have to give about the latest studies. Understanding your children will indeed help you to make the right parenting decisions. All the information that is disseminated should be evaluated according to God's Word and applied to individual circumstances by His Holy Spirit.

You can use all the worldly techniques available for toilet training, discipline, choosing a school and dealing with temper tantrums, and your child may do great. But in the long run, if you don't train your child in spiritual warfare, these exercises will be futile.

There is also plenty of garbage available in the world that could be detrimental to you and your child's mental and physical health. Some say that ungodly secular humanists in public schools and evil perpetrators that produce cartoons, toys and comic books are the enemies of our children. But the enemy is not a doll or a school teacher. Our fight should not be directed toward individuals or comic books. We battle the devil; the war is spiritual.

Always keep a clear view of your leader, Jesus Christ. Follow Him. Do what He commands. Likewise, remember your enemy is the devil, a cunning deviator who would like nothing more than your demise, physically and emotionally if possible, but most of all spiritually.

Prayer starter: Lord, help me to keep my eyes on You while I walk this earth, realizing that I am involved in a cosmic battle with the devil. Help me equip my child to wrestle not with flesh and blood but to be strong in You, Lord, so that she'll be able to stand against spiritual wickedness in high places.

DAY
133
"Stand firm then, with the belt of truth buckled around your waist" *(Eph. 6:14).*

Jesus says in John 14:6, "I am the way, the truth, and the life." Jesus is truth. By wearing the belt of truth, we've put on Jesus Christ.

Isaiah refers to the attributes of the Messiah in similar language: "Righteousness will be his belt and faithfulness the sash around his waist'' (11:5). A soldier for the Lord, therefore, has been made righteous by covering his sin with the blood of Jesus Christ.

Remember when you awaken to put on your belt of truth, a sash of faithfulness, available for you because Jesus paid the price for your sin.

Prayer starter: Lord, wrap around me the belt of truth, so that I might live my life cognizant of the fact that I am redeemed by Christ. I pray for this baby that she too will stand firm with truth buckled around her waist.

DAY 134

"...with the breastplate of righteousness in place" *(Eph. 6:14).*

The heart pumps life-giving blood to the rest of the body. During pregnancy, when the blood supply increases dramatically, the health of the heart is more important than ever. If the heart stops beating, both mother and baby die.

The Bible refers to the heart as the center for spiritual matters. The breastplate of righteousness serves as a bullet-proof vest to protect the inner person. Your spiritual heart made righteous through faith in Jesus pumps His life into all aspects of your being. So put on your breastplate!

You've got to "guard your heart, for it is the wellspring of life," Proverbs 4:23 says.

Prayer starter: Lord, thank You that through Jesus Christ I've been made righteous. Help me to wear the breastplate of righteousness, so that my spirit will be protected from the attacks of Satan. I pray for my baby, as his heart develops physically and spiritually, that You will bless him and instill within him a desire to seek righteousness through Christ.

DAY

135 "With your feet fitted with the readiness that comes from the gospel of peace" *(Eph. 6:15)*.

Put on your marching boots! You've got a message to take by foot, if necessary, to the rest of the world. Even though you're dressed as a soldier for battle, the message you bear is the gospel of peace, given to you from the Prince of Peace.

When Jesus gives the order, your feet have to be fit and ready to move. "Go and make disciples of all nations, baptizing them in the name of the Father and of the Son and of the Holy Spirit, and teaching them to obey everything I have commanded you," Jesus says in Matthew 28:19,20.

Properly fitted feet represent an offensive component of the armor. As you march forward, bearing the gospel of peace, many will hear and believe, and God's army will be strengthened.

Prayer starter: Lord, prepare me to march into all the earth, proclaiming Your good news. Give me boldness and confidence in You to carry the gospel of peace. I pray for my baby's feet that they would walk where You want them to walk and that he will be ready to share the love and peace of the Lord with his generation.

DAY

137 "In addition to all this, take up the shield of faith, with which you can extinguish all the flaming arrows of the evil one" *(Eph. 6:16)*.

Roman soldiers had leather shields that could be dipped in water to douse fiery arrows. The shield of faith immersed in living water can likewise extinguish the flaming arrows the devil shoots at us.

Living water is available to all through Jesus Christ. Jesus told the woman at the well in John 4:10, "If you knew the gift of God and who it is that asks for a drink, you would have asked him and he would have given you living water." When the devil shoots fear, doubt, worry or other negative thoughts at you to discourage and harm you, raise your shield of faith dripping with living water and the devil's lies will be doused.

Prayer starter: Father, strengthen my faith so that I can ward off the enemy's attack. Allow me to drink deeply of Your living water so that I'm filled to overflowing in my faith. I know that "greater is he that is in me than he that is in the world," according to 1 John 4:4. I pray for my baby that her faith in You will be strong and that she'll use her faith as a shield to protect herself from trouble in this world.

DAY
137 "Take the helmet of salvation" *(Eph. 6:17).*

There are two particularly vulnerable spots on the body that must be protected from physical harm: the heart and the head. Just as the breastplate protects the heart, the helmet protects the head. The head contains your brain, the center for your thoughts and actions. If the devil can influence your thought life, he can manipulate you.

Protect your mind with the helmet of salvation. Remember, you're a child of God, redeemed by Christ. "Now if we are children, then we are heirs—heirs of God and co-heirs with Christ," according to Romans 8:17. Our salvation means we stand to inherit the kingdom of God and eternal life.

When the devil attacks your thought life, put on your helmet of salvation. Rebuke the devil and his evil schemes so that your life remains pure. "Resist the devil, and he will flee from you" (James 4:7).

Prayer starter: Father, help me to put on my helmet of salvation, recognizing the fact that I'm Your child, a co-heir to Your kingdom with Your Son, Jesus Christ. When the devil attacks, bless my helmet of salvation, so that I won't be harmed. Bless my baby's developing mind. Prepare this child to don the helmet of salvation and to put on the mind of Christ.

DAY 138

"Take...the sword of the Spirit, which is the word of God" *(Eph. 6:17).*

The Word of God is "quick and powerful"; it is a living, active weapon that can knock down the enemy. When Jesus was tempted in the desert by the devil, He defeated Satan's attacks by quoting the Word of God.

When the enemy tries to plant little thoughts into your brain, counter him with Scripture.

"You're too stupid and inexperienced to be a mother," the devil may tell you.

"I can do everything through him who gives me strength," Philippians 4:13 says.

"Your baby's not going to be normal," the devil warns.

"I will fear no evil, for thou art with me," Psalm 23:4 says.

"You and your baby could die during childbirth," the devil may say.

"Fear not for I am with thee," the Lord tells His children over and over again in the Bible.

There are all kinds of new angles from which the devil will try to attack since you're carrying a new, unique individual. Be prepared: Carry the sword of the Spirit in your heart. Read your Bible every day and meditate on its meaning so that you can apply it to the circumstances you face.

Prayer starter: Lord, help me not only to read Your Word each day, but also to understand what You mean and use Your Word to fight the devil. I pray for my child that she will want to take up the sword of the Spirit, so that she'll be equipped to battle the enemy. Help me as a mother to read to her and set a good example for daily Bible reading.

DAY
139

"And pray in the Spirit on all occasions with all kinds of prayers and requests" *(Eph. 6:18).*

Surely Paul doesn't mean for us to pray "on all occasions." How can that be done? The Amplified Bible makes the command sound even more impossible: "Pray at all times—on every occasion, in every season...."

Keith Green wrote a song that begins to explain how this instruction from Paul can be accomplished. "Make My Life a Prayer to You," he sings to the Lord. If we offer ourselves as a living sacrifice to Him, we are His to do with as He likes. This requires us to remember whose we are. God-consciousness—an open prayer channel to and from Him—must be with us always.

As a soldier in God's army, prayer is another weapon in our warfare. Like a good soldier, we must listen to our leader's voice and obey. We also need to call upon Him through prayerful requests and supplication for help and strength to do the things that are impossible for us, knowing that nothing is impossible for Him.

Prayer starter: Lord, help me to be conscious of You, praying continually by making my life an offering of praise, thanksgiving, supplication, repentance, rejoicing, meditation and worship. I pray for my baby that he will learn to pray and use his prayer as a weapon to combat evil and further Your kingdom in his generation.

DAY
140

"Children, obey your parents in all things: for this is well pleasing unto the Lord" *(Col. 3:20, KJV).*

When I was pregnant with Holly, I was the morning announcer at WPLW radio. All of my regular listeners knew I was expecting, and many would send me words of encouragement. I remember one gift I received; it was an ABC learning book that taught the Scriptures to preschool children to go along with each letter of the alphabet. For the letter C the Scripture verse said, "Children, obey your parents for this is good." The accompanying illustration showed a little girl with a big smile on her face, picking up her toys.

I remember thinking, Will this baby ever be big enough to pick up toys with a big smile on her face? I figured it would be ages before I'd sit down to read the book to my child. I put it away to use at some future date.

But the time flew. Holly was less than a year old when I got out that book and began to read her the verses and show her the pictures. A few months later, before she could even talk, I remember saying, "Look, Holly, that little girl is obeying her mommy and it makes her happy. How do you look when you're happy?" She turned around and put a big smile on her face, imitating the little girl in the picture.

I don't know how much she understood about the message at that point, but I was *very* glad I had already begun to read to her.

Prayer starter: Lord, help me obey You, so that I'll be a good example for my children to obey their parents and ultimately You. Bless this baby with a teachable spirit and a heart to please and serve You.

DAY 141

"Greater love hath no man than this, that a man lay down his life for his friends" *(John 15:13, KJV).*

I don't get nauseated anymore except when riding in the car. If I drive, I'm fine. If not, I get pretty sick. With my hand securely on the wheel I can anticipate the bumps and turns in the road.

Thom doesn't mind. He understands and he encourages other people to let me drive, too. Recently Thom and I and our friend Randy were scheduled to sing at a church on the other side of town. We loaded our equipment into the small Japanese truck we borrowed and were about ready to leave when Thom's father pulled up to our house and said he'd love to come with us. The truck we were driving had little jump seats behind the front seats. They look big enough for a three-year-old to sit in.

When Thom announced to his father and Randy, both big guys, that I was going to drive and that they'd have to sit in these tiny seats, they stared at him in disbelief.

"You don't want her to get sick on all of us, do you?" he asked.

So Dad and Randy, the nice, kind men that they are, crawled into the cab and sat with their knees under their chins so that I could drive. Just as we left, it began to snow pretty hard and the driving was treacherous. Despite the uncomfortable ride, not one of the men complained. I'm so thankful for the wonderfully supportive men in my life!

Prayer starter: Lord, thank You for all the little blessings that help make this pregnancy easier. I pray my baby will have a servant's heart and love so great that he's willing to put others first. Thank You for the good role models this baby will have.

DAY 142

"A good name is better than precious ointment" (*Eccl. 7:1, KJV*).

Oh baby, what is your name? Are you strong and courageous? Gentle and happy? Musical? Pensive? Fearless? Meek? Shall I give you a name that reflects who you are? Or will you become what I've named you to be? Oh baby, what is your name?

For a boy, I'm thinking about the name Daniel Clark. Daniel means "God is my judge." This boy will walk uprightly, living his life according to the precepts of God. The prophet Daniel will serve as an excellent role model. Clark, my maiden name, means "scholar." With my father as his Clark connection, little Daniel will have a living example of a scholar who used his wisdom to build a successful career that provided stability for a happy household of seven.

If the baby's a girl, I want to name her Jeana Joy. Jeana comes from the same root as "John" which means "God is gracious." This baby will be the fourth child of a fourth child of a fourth child, so I want to name her for my mother, Jean. Mom is a very smart, talented lady and provides for me a great example for motherhood. I think most people who know her would agree that her outstanding characteristic is that she's full of fun, enjoys life and likes to spread her joy around to others.

Thom has held very strong opinions about the names of other children, but he says that so far he doesn't have a clear answer from God on this baby's name. He likes my two ideas, but he's very noncommittal.

Prayer starter: Lord, I pray that You'll make Your will clear to both Thom and me concerning the name of this baby. If You don't intend for us to name the baby either of the names we've considered, please tell us Your choice.

DAY 143

"The Lord, who stretches out the heavens, who lays the foundation of the earth and who forms the spirit of man within him..." *(Zech. 12:1).*

God not only designs our physical bodies, but the Bible says He also forms the spirit within us. He creates and breathes life into our inner selves. This spirit is created and begins to develop in the womb even while the physical body develops and grows.

John the Baptist, according to Luke 1:15, was "filled with the Holy Ghost, even from his mother's womb." I believe we can ask God to fill our babies with His Spirit even before they're born. Then we mothers while we're yet pregnant can nurture this growing child through our prayer and praise and through reading God's Word out loud. The little developing brain may not comprehend, but the spirit can still be blessed.

Prayer starter: Lord, I acknowledge You as the creator of all the aspects of my human life, physically, emotionally and spiritually. I believe You're creating the spirit within my baby, even as his body and mind develop. Fill my baby with Your Spirit so that just like John the Baptist he'll have the power to be used mightily by You.

DAY 144

"Therefore if any man be in Christ, he is a new creature: old things are passed away; behold, all things are become new" *(2 Cor. 5:17, KJV).*

The pure beauty and innocence of a newborn baby is a wonder to behold. I remember when Holly and David, then nearly four years and twenty months respectively, came to see Benjamin in the hospital a couple of hours after his birth. Holly couldn't take her eyes off him. I had never seen her so enthralled and excited. "Oh, Mommy, look at his little fingers! Oh, Mommy, look at his little ears!" She carefully examined and expressed admiration for all Benjamin's little body parts while David amused himself by playing with the switch that made the bed go up and down.

A spiritual newborn, like a brand new baby, has a pure beauty that comes through faith in Jesus Christ. The old person tainted by sin is washed clean and given the opportunity for a fresh start in life, no matter what he or she has done in the past.

As the babies within us grow and the date of delivery approaches, let's meditate on the thought that through Christ we've been made brand-new creatures, innocent and pure like a newborn, cleansed from sin. For just as we've been concentrating on asking God to perfect the physical bodies of our unborn babies, so we should invite Him to do a work in our lives. "For we are God's workmanship, created in Christ Jesus to do good works, which God prepared in advance for us to do" (Eph. 2:10).

Prayer starter: Lord, thank You for making me a new creation through Jesus Christ. I admit that, even as a new creature redeemed by Jesus, I make mistakes, I stumble and I fall. I pray You'll search me and show me my errors, so that I may repent and be washed clean once again. I acknowledge You as the One who recreated me to do good works for You. Help me to do the things that You want me to do.

DAY 145

"Your beauty should not come from outward adornment, such as braided hair and the wearing of gold jewelry and fine clothes. Instead, it should be that of your inner self, the unfading beauty of a gentle and quiet spirit, which is of great worth in God's sight" *(1 Pet. 3:3,4).*

I continually have my eye out for clothes that will enhance and accommodate my growing figure. While breezing through the local discount department store in search of a shower curtain, I spied a pair of cream-colored knit slacks that looked as if they'd be cute and comfortable throughout the duration of this pregnancy and also be great to wear after the baby is born.

I tried them on and they fit fine. The price was right, so I bought them. You can probably appreciate the joy in finding a comfortable pair of slacks that look dressy with a dressy blouse and casual with a casual top. The neutral color goes with everything. What a find! I know God was directing me to this treasure, more precious to a pregnant woman who's feeling not too attractive than a mink coat and an evening gown.

Yet, even as I thanked God for helping me find clothes that make me feel prettier, I got a little convicted. God cares more about my inner beauty—the appearance of my heart—than He does about my new cream-colored slacks. If I were as concerned about my inner beauty as I am about my outward appearance, I'm sure I would not mess up as much as I do.

Prayer starter: Lord, forgive me for my pride and vanity. Help me to look at my life the way You do and to develop my inner beauty and strength more than my outward appearance. I do thank You for providing me with clothes to wear at this time, and I vow to keep these material goods in the proper perspective.

DAY 146

"My grace is sufficient for you, for my power is made perfect in weakness" *(2 Cor. 12:9).*

Considering that parenthood may be the most important job assignment God gives us, you'd think we would receive better training. Teachers serve as student teachers before tackling a classroom single-handedly. Pilots train beside experts before attempting a solo flight. Doctors serve as residents before graduating from medical school. But mothers and fathers are required to get on-the-job training. It's a wonder any first children survive!

I remember when Holly was about a month old. She was a very peaceful baby during the day. At night she was peaceful, too, as long as she was being held, preferably by an adult who walked around singing to her. One night, while trying to interest Holly in nursing instead of a midnight stroll, Thom suggested I find the pacifier someone had given to me at a baby shower. The thought had never occurred to me. No one ever discipled me in the use of pacifiers as a means to find peace. I quickly found the pacifier, took it out of the package, washed it and stuck it in Holly's mouth. She instantly began to suck and stopped crying. She fell asleep.

I know some people don't believe in pacifiers, so be sure to study the subject before you decide to try one. David never liked them. He sucked his thumb instead. Benjamin did take a pacifier. Babies have a natural instinct to suck that is not always satisfied through eating alone. I had to find this out for each baby through trial and error.

Trials and errors. That's how rookies become parents. But we have hope because in our weakness God is strong. God knows we don't know how to parent our children perfectly. That forces us to look to Him. For every individual child, He teaches us step-by-step how to be a parent.

Prayer starter: Lord, thank You for Your all-sufficient grace. I confess my weakness, particularly in parenting this baby with whom You've blessed me and my husband. In our weakness perfect Your power in us.

DAY 147

"Nehemiah said, 'Go and enjoy choice food and sweet drinks, and send some to those who have nothing prepared. This day is sacred to our Lord. Do not grieve, for the joy of the Lord is your strength' " *(Neh. 8:10).*

Nehemiah instructed the people to celebrate during the Feast of Tabernacles, a time set apart for thanksgiving for the harvest and commemorating the Israelis' time spent in tents as they crossed the wilderness. This was not your everyday party. This was a special time for celebrating the goodness of God.

It was with this inspirational mandate from Nehemiah in mind that Thom and I recently sought out a pizza shop in Pittsburgh that is highly acclaimed for its tasty, extravagant pizzas. The homemade dough is thick and fresh, piled with the finest meats and cheeses and sweet peppers and onions. We went there recently without our other children to have a night out together, enjoying each other's company. The food was terrific—so rich and filling we were forced to bring some home so our stomachs wouldn't burst.

We need to set aside a time to rejoice, feast and have fun. If most of the time we carefully watch our diets and exercise self-control in our eating and drinking habits, we can afford an evening of celebration. When the baby arrives, it will be more difficult to get out on a date with your husband, so plan a few special evenings to rejoice in God's goodness before the baby comes.

Prayer starter: Lord, thank You for helping us set aside special times to feast, rejoice and enjoy Your goodness. I pray You'll bless the fruit of my womb and bless my life with the fruit of Your Spirit. Thank You for reminding me that I have strength through the joy I find in You.

DAY 148

"Because thy lovingkindness is better than life, my lips shall praise thee. Thus will I bless thee while I live: I will lift up my hands in thy name" *(Ps. 63:3,4, KJV).*

While singing a chorus using this passage as its lyrics, I suddenly stop to wonder, How can loving-kindness be better than life? All I can figure is this: God is love, the Bible says. He is also the life-giver. Combining love and life is better than life without God's love.

"For God so loved the world, that He gave His only begotten Son, that whoever believes in Him should not perish, but have eternal life," John 3:16 says. God loves me and gives me life eternally because I believe in Jesus. I can have love and life! Hallelujah! My lips do praise Him, and with joy I reach up to my heavenly Father in thanks for my life and the precious life that is growing inside me.

Prayer starter: Father, thank You for Your loving-kindness that allows me to have life through Jesus Christ. I praise and thank You. Bless my baby with lips that will sing Your praises and hands that reach out to worship You and to do Your will.

DAY
149

"But whosoever drinketh of the water that I shall give him shall never thirst; but the water that I shall give him shall be in him a well of water springing up into everlasting life" *(John 4:14, KJV).*

Holly and I have decided that we're going to help each other drink eight glasses of water each day.

"It's hard, Mom. I can't drink that much water," she tells me.

"Drinking plenty of water cleans your insides, just as soap and water clean your outsides," I remind Holly (and myself).

Jesus offered the woman at the well living water to satisfy her thirst and to cleanse her from the inside out. This woman had been looking for love in all the wrong places. She had had five husbands and at least one live-in lover. Perhaps she was used and abused by all these guys. Whatever her circumstances she jumped at the chance to find real love through Jesus, to drink from the eternal spring He offered and be washed of her sins.

While I'm on my drink-plenty-of-water campaign, I try to remember the living water Jesus offers and keep my eyes on eternity.

Prayer starter: Lord, thank You that my soul does not need to be parched and dry, because Jesus Christ satisfied my thirst with water which springs up into everlasting life. I pray for my child that You will instill in her a thirst for righteousness.

How do you feel? Has God revealed anything special to you about yourself or your child? What are your greatest concerns at this time? Does your doctor have any words of advice? Have you been praying for the fruit of self-control to grow in your life? What do you like to wear? Have you bought maternity clothes yet?

Thy Wife—A Fruitful Vine?

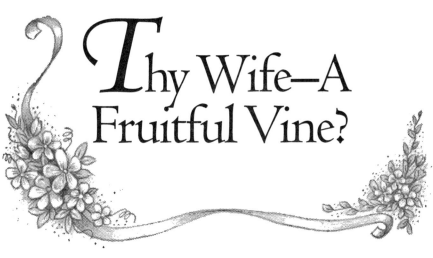

DAYS 150–179

MONTH SIX This month the baby will grow an inch or two, averaging around fourteen inches and weighing just over a pound. Buds for permanent teeth come in, eyelashes form, and eyelids separate. The fingernails grow to the end of the fingers. The baby has a strong grip and can cry, suck, make a fist, kick and turn somersaults in the womb. Can you feel those acrobatics?

You will be putting on weight fairly regularly now, as the baby begins to fill out. This is a good month to make sure your loose ends are tied on the job, at home and in preparing for the baby's physical needs.

Prayer starter: Lord, guard my baby from any harm as Your developmental process continues inside the womb. Continue to prepare me, Your daughter, to be the mother You want me to be to this baby.

DAY 150

"Thy wife shall be as a fruitful vine by the sides of thine house..." *(Ps. 128:3, KJV).*

Bright green ivy adorns an old stone church near my house, framing the stained glass windows and polished oak doors. The vine gives the church a warm, happy look that contrasts with the cold gray stones. Was this the type of vine the psalmist envisioned? One glance in the mirror confirms that I look like a fruitful vine all right. But it's not ivy or even a grapevine. I look like a watermelon vine with one ripe, round melon right in the middle. God is literally blessing the fruit of my womb. I pray that as I bring this baby to term He'll also bless me with the fruit of His Spirit.

Prayer starter: Lord, thank You for blessing my husband and me with fruit, this child, the physical result of our love for one another. I pray You'll continue to bless my whole family with the fruit of Your Spirit, the result of our love for You.

DAY 151

"But the fruit of the Spirit is...kindness" *(Gal. 5:22).*

I saw kindness personified at the local laundromat. A pregnant mother with beads of sweat on her brow leaned over a laundry basket full of dirty clothes. Her tiny son, probably around two years old, was sitting on the washing machine. He threw his arms around his mother's bent head, pulled her face up to his face, then gently wiped the perspiration from her forehead and gave her a kiss. This child, who displayed such a tender act of kindness, surely is treated with gentle kindness.

The dictionary defines "kind" as "having gentleness, tenderness or goodness of heart." A kind person is a nice person, one who listens more than she talks; esteems others as better than herself; bakes two pies instead of one so she can give one away. Kindness is more than a state of mind. Kindness that is harvested as a fruit of the Spirit requires action.

Ephesians 4:32 is one of the first verses my children memorized because they've heard it over and over again. "Be ye kind one to another, tenderhearted, forgiving one another, even as God for Christ's sake hath forgiven you" (KJV).

Most people can muster up enough human kindness to get by on. God's kindness requires us to be tender to everyone, to be forgiving, because He forgave us. Psalm 18:50 says, "He shows unfailing kindness to his anointed." God's kindness doesn't fail. Isaiah 54:8 says, "With everlasting kindness I will have compassion on you." God's kindness is everlasting and full of compassion.

Jesus showed kindness, mercy and compassion on people through the miracles He performed. His miraculous acts—restoring sight to the blind, raising the dead, healing the sick—not only demonstrated His power, but they also displayed His kindness. Jesus showed He loved the people through acts of kindness.

Prayer starter: Lord, help me to be full of the fruit of Your kindness. Teach me to be kind and tenderhearted. Let kindness literally take root in my heart. Bless my baby with a kind heart. Let her friends and family some day say, "She is kind."

DAY
152
"If anyone wishes to come after Me, let him deny himself, and take up his cross, and follow Me" *(Matt. 16:24, NAS).*

A new mother recently told me, "I've been a Christian a long time, but I don't think I really understood 'denying myself' until I became a mother. When the baby's hungry, tired, wet or wanting to play, I forget my needs and tend to her."

Jesus is the example of servanthood. He laid down His life for His friends, denying Himself. He calls us to do likewise, which is a bit more challenging than losing sleep to change and feed an infant.

This verse starts with a big "if." God doesn't force us to follow Him. He gives us the choice to say yes or no to Him. If we decide to follow, denying ourselves, He tells us to pick up our cross. Some people interpret this to mean dealing with the drudgery of life, suffering for His sake. Maybe now as our babies are growing larger and larger, some will be tempted to say, "This is just our cross to bear."

I don't believe this verse teaches that at all. The cross for Christ was His destiny, the job the Father sent Him to do. My cross is the work God has given me. Right now that includes caring for three small children while I carry a fourth inside of me and writing these devotions to encourage other expectant mothers. These "crosses"—divine assignments—bring me tremendous joy.

This joy lines up with Scripture, for Christ says in John 15:11, "These things have I spoken unto you, that my joy might remain in you, and that your joy might be full" (KJV).

Prayer starter: Lord, I want to follow You. Help me to deny myself, not only so that I'll be a good mother, but so that I'll be the kind of servant You want me to be to my family, friends and neighbors. Show me my cross, so that I can joyfully do the work You want me to do.

DAY 153

"But you will receive power when the Holy Spirit comes on you..." *(Acts 1:8).*

In Pittsburgh, streetcars continue to play a vital role in public transportation. Ever since I was a little girl I was fascinated with the trolley cars, whose big steel wheels follow a precise path, forged in the brick and concrete streets of our city. The power for the trolley comes from a cable up above.

My life used to follow a path forged by my own decisions. Somewhere along the line, I accepted Jesus Christ as my Savior. His Spirit filled me and gave me power from on high. Now through God's Spirit I'm able to stay on track.

Prayer starter: O God, fill me anew with Your Spirit. Give me the power today to do what You want me to do. Touch my baby with Your Spirit, too, O Lord. Keep Your hand upon her as she grows.

DAY 154

"A student is not above his teacher, but everyone who is fully trained will be like his teacher" *(Luke 6:40).*

The children in our church were preparing to present a praise processional. With joyful singing they practiced marching down the aisle, moving their hands with military motions. When five-year-old Joanna, the littlest child in the processional, could not coordinate her hands with the beat, her teacher put her hands over Joanna's until she learned the movements correctly. With this accomplished, Joanna testified to her class, "I couldn't do it, but teacher put her hands over mine. Now I can do it. Look!"

Jesus Christ is our teacher. As prospective parents, we have so much to learn. If we go to Him with childlike faith and admit our shortcomings, He gently puts His hands over ours and shows us what to do.

The more we study the character of Christ and learn to be like Him, the better equipped we become to take on any task this world has to offer.

Prayer starter: Lord, teach me Your ways. Help me to become more and more like You every day. Help me teach my child all I know about You, so that he can become a teacher, too.

DAY 155

"I, the Lord your God, am a jealous God, punishing the children for the sin of the fathers to the third and fourth generation of those who hate me, but showing love to a thousand generations who love me and keep my commandments" *(Ex. 20:5,6).*

One woman I know expressed concern for her unborn child, fearing that God would punish the baby for the mother's and grandparents' sins. "I sowed a lot of wild oats before I came to know the Lord," she said. "So did Mom and Dad. The Bible says you reap what you sow. I'm afraid my baby's going to have to pay the penalty for my stupid mistakes."

145

This is unscriptural thinking. Jesus paid the penalty for all of our sin. God loves us so much He sent His Son to die, so that those who believe in Him would not have to pay the price for their sin. If you love and obey the Lord, He promises to show His love to a thousand generations.

"There is therefore now no condemnation to them which are in Christ Jesus," the Bible says in Romans 8:1 (KJV). There is no reason to walk around feeling guilty for sins that have been forgiven. If you have been raised in a family that perhaps even for generations has been caught up in a cycle of ungodly living that perpetuates itself from parent to child, parent to child, it is possible to break that cycle. God can help you if you submit your life to Him. He will give you the power to take an axe to the root cause of sin in your life and end the effects of that bad root once and for all.

Prayer starter: Lord, I believe that, even though in the lineage of my family in the past several generations there has been sin, I have been set free from paying the penalty for that sin because Christ died for me. Lord, I receive Your forgiveness for my past mistakes. I pray the seeds of sin I've sown will suffer crop failure, because they're gone, wiped clean, unable to grow. I love and want to obey You, Lord, and I receive Your promise to show love to this baby and her succeeding generations.

DAY 156

"Taste and see that the Lord is good; blessed is the man who takes refuge in him" *(Ps. 34:8).*

Taste buds are cropping up inside the baby's cheeks and on his tongue. Will my baby enjoy his food, relishing the crunch of a crisp carrot and savoring the sweet goodness of a baked apple? Or will he prefer the crunch of potato chips and the sweetness of a candy bar?

So far, my little ones respond positively when I explain which foods are good for their growing bodies and which foods don't do them much good. Just as I hope and pray that my children will choose to eat food that will help their physical growth, I also pray that they'll have a taste for good spiritual food that will help their spirits grow in the things of God. My children will not develop healthy, godly characteristics if they receive a steady diet of television shows and comic books. But the little ones who taste and see that the Lord is good will acquire a hunger and thirst for righteousness. These children will feed on God's Word and develop strong hearts and minds.

Prayer starter: Father, as my baby's taste buds develop, I pray that she will have a taste for healthy foods that will strengthen her physical body. I also pray that this baby develops a hunger for the things of God, so that when she tastes and sees that You are good, Lord, she will be blessed, putting her trust in You.

DAY 157

"There are six things the Lord hates, seven that are detestable to him" *(Prov. 6:16).*

Pregnancy is such a happy, positive time. So far, throughout these devotions, I've tried to emphasize the joyful, life-giving, encouragement and special love God pours on expectant mothers during this precious time.

But I'd also like to meditate for the next few days on what the Lord says He hates, so that as mothers we can avoid these sins and pray that our babies will avoid them as well.

Prayer starter: Lord, teach me to flee from evil and cling to what is good. Help me to avoid the things You hate and teach my child to do the same.

DAY 158

"The Lord hates...haughty eyes" *(Prov. 6:16,17).*

Haughty means "proud and arrogant." I can think of more than just a few women who wear their pregnancies with pride. Look at Leah and Rachel, Jacob's wives, who competed in giving children to their husband (see Gen. 30). Leah had four boys, while Rachel had none, so Rachel gave her servant to her husband to bear children for her. Rachel's servant had two sons, so then Leah gave her servant to her husband, and that servant had two sons. Leah had two more sons and a daughter, then Rachel had two sons. These women, who were sisters, were jealous of one another. Leah envied Rachel because Jacob loved Rachel more. Rachel was jealous of Leah because of the many children she bore for Jacob. When they were pregnant, more than likely, both of them walked around with proud, haughty eyes.

Indeed, children are gifts. But the Father blesses both the godly and the ungodly with these precious children. We should not esteem ourselves higher than others during pregnancy; we ought to heed Paul's instructions to the Philippians to "esteem others better than ourselves." Psalm 18:27 says, "You save the humble but bring low those whose eyes are haughty."

Prayer starter: Father, forgive me for my pride. Help me to boast in You and the work Christ does in me, not in myself. I pray for my baby's eyes that they would not be haughty, but that they would be focused on Jesus.

DAY
159 "The Lord hates...a lying tongue" *(Prov. 6:16,17).*

Pregnant women may be tempted to lie in a variety of ways.

There's the direct lie: "I gained twenty pounds when I was pregnant." (Add a dozen and a half more pounds and you find the truth.)

There's the indirect lie: "Honey, what did you eat for dinner?" your husband asks. "I had a cheese sandwich and a salad," you reply, not mentioning that you also ate a bag of potato chips with dip, six chocolate chip cookies and a hot fudge sundae.

There's the pregnant lady's lazy lie, designed to win her husband's attention and sympathy: "Sweetheart, I don't feel real well. Could you please make dinner tonight? One more chore will add too much physical and emotional stress on me and your unborn child."

Whatever the variety, God hates lies. Psalm 34:13 says, "Keep your tongue from evil and your lips from speaking lies."

Prayer starter: Father, help me to speak only truthful words that bring glory and honor to Your name. I pray for my baby as she develops that You would bless her tongue to speak truthfully.

DAY 160

"The Lord hates…hands that shed innocent blood" *(Prov. 6:16,17).*

There is none more innocent than an unborn baby, a child God ordains and forms, growing safely in his or her mother's womb. God loves each woman and her baby. But He hates hands that shed innocent blood.

The abortionists and our society which condones abortion will have to stand before God accounting for the thousands upon thousands of innocent lives whose blood has been shed.

Prayer starter: Father, forgive us for standing by, allowing innocent blood to be shed in our nation. We lift up to You the women who are considering abortion. Move by Your Spirit to show them and the world that You hate hands that shed innocent blood. I pray for my baby's hands that they would be clean, used only to do good works for You.

DAY 161

"The Lord hates…a heart that devises wicked schemes, feet that are quick to rush into evil" *(Prov. 6:16,18).*

Before your feet can run to do evil, your mind has devised the wicked scheme. Let's look at a totally fictitious scenario. A pregnant woman, who has quit smoking because she knows cigarettes are bad for her and the baby, is tempted one day to smoke. Instead of casting down the tempting thought, she indulges in it a little bit, wondering if perhaps there's a leftover cigarette in the bottom of her purse. She looks to no avail so she searches throughout the house. Finding nary a butt, she devises a scheme: Instead of facing a store clerk who might add to her guilt, she decides to walk to the corner bar to buy some cigarettes out of the machine. Her feet are all too willing to go along with the scheme. In the bar she gets into more trouble by indulging in an unplanned drink or two. Hearts that plan evil schemes and feet quick to rush into trouble often work together.

The evil starts with a thought. If we've got our eyes on Jesus and are continually looking to Him to guide and direct us, He will direct our path.

Prayer starter: Lord, search my heart and show me any wicked schemes that I may have devised. Forgive me for any plans I make that do not line up with Your Word and Your perfect will for my life. Help me to avoid evil by keeping my feet walking in Your light. I pray for my baby's heart that it would be pure before You and that, as she grows, You'll help keep her feet on the path that leads to life.

DAY 162

"The Lord hates...a false witness who pours out lies" *(Prov. 6:16,19).*

A false witness is one who is slanderous, who lies about another. Slanderous statements can arise through misunderstandings and gossip, or simply when one person fabricates lies to hurt or discredit another person.

God hates this! Sometimes we think it's OK to repeat slanderous rumors if it involves people we don't know, but it's not.

I've found a good antidote for the poison of slander. Turn Philippians 4:8 around to say, "Whatever's not nice, whatever's not kind, whatever's false and disgusting, keep your mind (and your mouth) off of these things!"

Prayer starter: Lord, forgive me if I ever have slandered or received a false witness concerning another person. Help me always to live righteously and to point others to righteous living as well.

DAY 163

"The Lord hates...a man who stirs up dissension among brothers" *(Prov. 6:16,19).*

If you do or say something to cause trouble among people who have a loving relationship with one another, you're stirring dissension among brothers (and/or sisters).

"But you don't know how Betty has hurt me!" a woman recently cried to me about our mutual friend. She proceeded to tell me how she had been hurt, causing me to have a pretty low opinion of Betty, if the story was true.

"Go tell Betty how you feel about what she's done," I told her. Now how do I face Betty, not wanting to get more involved than I am?

The Bible says in Matthew 18:15, "If your brother sins against you, go and show him his fault, just between the two of you. If he listens to you, you have won your brother over." It seems that much dissension among brothers and sisters in the church arises when people do not handle conflicts in a biblical manner. If we have a problem with someone, that person is about the hundredth person to find out about it as we bounce the details off of eager ears. This causes dissension.

We need to keep our conflicts as simple as possible. Direct confrontation is hard, and it must be done in love with much prayer.

Prayer starter: Lord, help me to be a peacemaker, not one who causes strife and dissension. Bless my baby to be a person who is a blessing to his brothers and sisters, not a troublemaker.

DAY
164
"And we know that in all things God works for the good of those who love him, who have been called according to his purpose" *(Rom. 8:28).*

Annie found out, while she was six months pregnant with her third child, that her husband was having an affair. All parties involved called themselves Christians, which somehow made it even harder for Annie to accept. Not only was her faith in her husband shattered, but her faith in God wavered as well. Her husband repented, as did the "other woman," but Annie could not piece her life back together. She felt unattractive, unwanted and unloved. Her low self-esteem made it difficult for her husband, who was an emotional wreck as well, to try to rekindle their troubled marriage.

"Through all of this," Annie told me, "I clung with one thin thread to the hope that God could work in these circumstances and make something beautiful out of the ashes of our lives.''

The restoration process has been a slow uphill battle, but Annie seems to be close to the crest of the hill. She still can see the low points in the valley, but her eyes are set on the hope that is before her. She's still married, the children are thriving, and she only occasionally suffers from depression.

Sometimes seemingly insurmountable problems happen to us. Being pregnant does not make us immune to the attacks of the enemy. We may be an even greater target for the devil as we bring a new innocent life into the world.

But whatever terrible circumstances we're in, God says He is in the midst, working through the problems of those who love Him and are called according to His purposes.

Prayer starter: Lord, You know those areas of my life where I'm struggling. You know better than I do the mountains and obstacles that have appeared in the path I walk. I trust You to work out all things for my good, because I love You and I'm called according to Your purposes. Bless my baby as he goes with me through the ups and downs of this pregnancy. Protect him from evil.

DAY
165

"There is no fear in love. But perfect love drives out fear, because fear has to do with punishment. The man who fears is not made perfect in love" *(1 John 4:18).*

One woman told me that when she was pregnant with her third child she was overwhelmed with fear. The fear had taken root through several different circumstances. The first was the fact that she had an abortion prior to her conversion, and she still dealt with guilt. Even though she believed God had forgiven her, she could not forgive herself, and she feared her unborn child would somehow be punished. She also feared because her previous pregnancy had been long and very difficult. She was told that if she hadn't been in a hospital, she and the baby could have died. If she allowed her mind to dwell on these thoughts, she became terrified. She confessed her fears and feelings to her husband, and together they prayed for her and the new baby. God quickened 1 John 4:18 to her mind, and over and over again she meditated on the fact that "perfect love drives out fear." She told me she thought about God's perfect love for her as she prayed.

Her labor and delivery lasted one hour. "I didn't have *time* to be afraid," she testified joyfully. The baby weighed nine and a half pounds, more than the previous child who doctors said was too big to deliver safely. God not only delivered a precious baby into the world, He also delivered this woman from fear and guilt!

Prayer starter: Father, I thank You for Your perfect love, and I receive Your love into my life. I know Your love cannot dwell with fear and that Your love actually drives out fear. Help me remember, when I am afraid, that You love me and that You love my child and want only what's best for us. I pray for my baby that he, too, will know Your perfect love and never have to fear.

DAY
166 "Therefore, prepare your minds for action" *(1 Pet. 1:13).*

God wonderfully made our bodies to bear children! Even in the earlier months of pregnancy, you may have experienced mild contractions. By now, these Braxton-Hicks contractions (so named because Braxton-Hicks was the first to notice them) can be felt sporadically tightening and softening the uterine muscle. Be happy when you feel these contractions. It means your body's exercising so that the muscle will be good and strong on labor day; this is your uterus preparing physically to deliver the baby. Think about this when the "practice" contractions come. Take a deep, cleansing breath. Relax. Focus your thoughts on the peace of God until the contraction is over. You can prepare your mind for action!

Prayer starter: Father, thank You for creating my body to bear children. Just as my muscles prepare to give birth, help me put on the mind of Christ so that I'll be prepared mentally to have this baby.

DAY 167

"Trust in the Lord with all your heart and lean not on your own understanding; in all your ways acknowledge him, and he will make your paths straight" *(Prov. 3:5,6).*

"How long should I plan to work?" a pregnant friend asked me. Inside or outside of the home, this is a question that must be answered on an individual basis according to each woman's unique needs and circumstances. When I was carrying Holly, I worked a four-hour daily shift as a radio announcer. I scheduled my replacement to start on my due date, because I felt great and would have been bored had I left the job sooner. She was born three weeks later, and I don't recall ever getting bored. I was working in our *Expression* office laying out an issue of the magazine when I went into labor with Benjamin.

Those whose jobs are more strenuous or have to sit or stand too much should consider taking leave earlier. In Great Britain, the twenty-ninth week of pregnancy is the accepted time to take off from work.

God cares about the intimate details of our lives. When we put our trust in Him and acknowledge Him as the ruler, humbling ourselves and deferring to His guidance, He directs our paths. Trust God; seek His guidance. He will show you what type of activities to engage in over the next few months—and the rest of Your life if you allow Him.

Prayer starter: Father, I put my trust in You with all of my heart, and I acknowledge You as my Lord. I will follow where You lead me. Show me what to do regarding the work I do in and out of my home as it relates to this pregnancy and my baby. Confirm Your direction for me to my husband, too, so that we may stand united in Your will for our lives. I pray my baby, too, will put his trust in You, so that even his earliest decisions will be made according to Your plan for him.

DAY 168

"Blessed are the peacemakers: for they shall be called the children of God" *(Matt. 5:9, KJV).*

154

Where does the world's bloodiest daily violence take place? I don't think it's in the villages of Central America, the streets of Belfast or in the war-torn Middle East. Although these areas are well-acquainted with war, the violence does not go on all day every day. I believe the scene for the worst massacre of our age is in the antiseptic atmosphere of our hospitals, clinics and doctors' offices where thousands of unborn children are ripped, sucked, chemically burned, and mutilated in their mothers' wombs. Places that were built to bring healing have been turned into slaughter houses because society condones the killing of the innocent who should have safety and peace within their mother. Christ calls us to be peacemakers, people whom He uses to take His peace into conflict. A woman faces a crisis with her unborn child when that child is unwanted. It's our job, as peacemakers, to help the woman come to a peaceful, loving solution to what she views as a problem. The peaceful alternatives to abortion are as varied as the situations of crisis pregnancies.

How will we ever solve the conflicts of nation against nation if we as a society cannot come to a peaceful solution for unwanted pregnancy? It's clear that God ordains life. We have no right as an individual or a society to terminate life for the sake of convenience. That is not how Jesus handles conflict.

If you or someone you know is experiencing an unwanted pregnancy, know that God loves every mother and every child. He has a plan for both of you, or He would not have created you. Seek God concerning His perfect will for you and your baby. He will provide a loving, peaceful solution for your conflict.

Prayer starter: Father, I pray for every woman who is experiencing an unwanted pregnancy. Please pour out Your love on them. Let them know You have a special place in Your kingdom for each individual You form in the womb. Father, if any who have had an abortion are reading this, pour Your Spirit upon them, allowing them to find forgiveness and healing in You. Help us, Your church, to be peacemakers, available to serve our sisters who need help in continuing their pregnancies and raising their children.

DAY 169

"Have nothing to do with godless myths and old wives' tales; rather, train yourself to be godly" *(1 Tim. 4:7)*.

Have you noticed how many childbirth experts there are in the world? Many women *and* men are only too anxious to share stories. Beware! Tales that do not line up with God's Word should be ignored.

Sitting in a revival meeting listening to a world-renowned evangelist recently, I was disgusted and appalled to hear this man retell a metaphor that I think the devil himself spreads to put fear into pregnant woman. For a cheap laugh, the preacher compared childbirth to having one's lips stretched and pulled over his or her head. Many of the people in the congregation laughed. I excused my obviously pregnant body to the ladies' room.

In the ladies' room, a pregnant teenager, who looked close to her due date, sat crying. Holding my own round belly, I asked her if I could do anything to help. She said no, so I prayed silently for her and any of the other pregnant women in the crowd.

This experience made me mad! The source of fear is located in hell. God created our bodies wonderfully. We are designed to reproduce. Through Jesus Christ we are set free from the curse of sin. Sisters, we should not listen to old wives' tales, rather train ourselves to be godly.

Prayer starter: Lord, I pray for the men and women of this world, that You would teach them about the beauty of Your creation, that they would not mock You or be used of the devil to instill fear into pregnant women. Father, give me a teachable heart so that I will train myself in godliness, holding all I see and hear up to the light of Your Word, casting down the myths and the ungodly.

DAY 170

"I called upon the Lord in distress: the Lord answered me and set me in a large place" *(Ps. 118:5, KJV)*.

The bank decided to reconsider our loan application before foreclosing on the large house we wanted to buy. At first, I couldn't believe it. I had stopped thinking about the house, believing the Lord had closed the door. In my heart I had released the need for more living space into God's hands and was waiting to see what would happen.

We provided the bank with the additional information they wanted, worked out some details with the help of family, and guess what? We close in one month! I'll be able to bring my new baby home to a nursery set up for him or her exclusively. I'm so excited I can hardly wait. Thank You, Jesus! Now all we have to do is sell or rent our little house.

I don't know what needs you may have for your baby. But my advice is, give those needs to the Lord. Over and over again He proves that He provides all our needs according to His riches in glory.

Prayer starter: Father, I know in my heart that You provide for all of my needs. I thank You and praise You that again You've taught me to trust in You, to have faith to believe that You answer prayer. Lord, let my life be a testimony of Your goodness and love to the baby I'm carrying. Help me teach my child to turn to You for her provision.

DAY
171 "What have they seen in thine house?" *(2 Kin. 20:15, KJV).*

Thoughts of moving to a large house with plenty of closets, shelves and storage space fill my mind as I glance around my crowded kitchen. Plastic containers fall on my head when I open the cupboard door above the sink. Everything that can be hung—from mixing spoons and graters to skillets, strainers, pots and potato mashers—hang on a pegboard that covers one wall.

What do people see in my house? Right now they see disaster! Dirty windows (pregnant women shouldn't climb ladders, right?), toys strewn from room to room, and floors that cry out, "Scrub me! Scrub me!" greet the eyes of my visitors.

Yet I continually have visitors. I see my house as a happy home. It's a peaceful place, even while it looks like a battle zone. When the children are loud, they normally make joyful noises, not quarrelsome sounds. I hope that visitors see the love of the Lord in my home, despite the state of housekeeping.

I hope and pray that my baby will find love, peace and joy in the home Thom and I have established, not chaos and confusion.

Prayer starter: Help me, Lord, to prioritize my life according to Your plans. Help me to teach my children that there's a time to play games and a time to put toys away. Teach me to be better organized, especially with a baby on the way, so that I'll have a household that's not only a fun place full of love and peace, but also a tidy home that's full of Your joy.

DAY
172

"When I was a child, I used to speak as a child, think as a child, reason as a child; when I became a man, I did away with childish things" *(1 Cor. 13:11, NAS).*

My mother has an amazing gift that endears children to her. She understands the childish mind so well that she's a continual source of fun and entertainment. She sows her life and love into children by giving her time and energy to invent treasure hunts and games, to act out stories and to have a good time in general.

During a recent visit, Mom decided we would act out a story, then proceeded to assign the parts with the available actors. While I pretended to be a tree full of apples—waiting for Benjamin, the monkey, to ride on top of Holly, the elephant, to take apples to David, the wise old owl—the thought occurred to me that mothers really need to learn how to be children again. We use this knowledge not to act like children but so that we can better understand our kids and meet their needs.

As we prepare to have babies, we should ask the Lord to give us all the insight we need to be the best mothers we possibly can be to our children.

Prayer starter: Lord, I come to You humbly, as Your little child, admitting my shortcomings and ignorance regarding motherhood. But, Lord, I trust that You who ordained motherhood will prepare me to be the mother You want me to be. Help me remember how to think as a child, so that I'll be able to understand and serve my children.

DAY

173 "Lord, teach us to pray" *(Luke 11:1, KJV)*.

This request by one of His disciples prompted Jesus to teach what we know as "the Lord's prayer," found in Luke 11:2-4. This prayer provides the prototype of how we're to pray. I memorized this prayer in first grade during the days when it was OK to acknowledge God in public schools.

Prayer is gone from public schools, so parents who want their children to pray must teach them. The Lord's prayer, short and relatively simple, can be memorized easily by preschool children. We also teach our children to pray through example. Family devotions provide an opportunity for parents to share all kinds of spiritual lessons for their children.

My cousin gave me an idea for encouraging children to pray. It has become a big hit in our family. We have a prayer basket that contains index cards the children have colored with the names of various relatives and friends. During prayer time, each family member picks a card at random and prays for that person. The children delight in finding out for whom they're to pray.

Prayer starter: Our Father which art in heaven, Hallowed be thy name. Thy kingdom come. Thy will be done, as in heaven, so in earth. Give us day by day our daily bread. And forgive us our sins; for we also forgive every one that is indebted to us. And lead us not into temptation; but deliver us from evil. Help me, Lord, to pray and to teach my little one to pray.

DAY

174 "All scripture is God-breathed and is useful for teaching, rebuking, correcting and training in righteousness, so that the man of God may be thoroughly equipped for every good work" *(2 Tim. 3:16,17)*.

My faith is built when I hear good preaching and teaching. I hear good messages in church, and I also hear them on radio and television.

God doesn't want me to be simply a "hearer" of His Word. He wants me to be a "doer" too.

To do God's will, I have to know His will. To know His will, I must read His Word. All alone with the Bible, I receive God's Word that equips *me* to teach, rebuke, correct and train myself and others in righteousness.

If I only attended the electronic church, I wouldn't be able to interact with the rest of the Lord's body. I may be equipped to teach and train, but sitting in my living room in front of the television I'd have no one to share with.

As God forms little bodies in our wombs, He's also forming little souls and spirits. As mothers, we are the first preachers and teachers these babies will hear. We must, as Paul continues in his second letter to Timothy, "preach the Word; be prepared in season and out of season; correct, rebuke and encourage—with great patience and careful instruction" (4:2).

Prayer starter: Lord, as I prepare to give birth, further prepare me to be the mother You want me to be. Give me wisdom and discernment as I read Your Word, so that I'll be equipped to train, teach and correct my child.

DAY 175

"Weeping may remain for a night, but rejoicing comes in the morning" *(Ps. 30:5).*

As the baby grows, I find myself getting more and more tired as the day wears on. In mid-afternoon I feel strong enough to conquer the world. But by the time the children are in bed and I finally want to dig into some new project, I'm too tired. Fatigue inevitably clouds my perception, and I either give up in frustration or sit down and cry.

After a good night's sleep, I'm a new woman! The psalmist must have known the feeling I'm talking about when he wrote: "Your troops will be willing on your day of battle. Arrayed in holy majesty, from the womb of the dawn you will receive the dew of your youth" (Ps. 110:3).

Just as new life will come from my womb, so does the morning bring revitalization to my tired body. In the morning I can rejoice and go forth to conquer the world. We pregnant women need to get plenty of good sleep and rest so that we have strength during the day to do the work the Lord wants us to do. Each dawn brings a new day full of opportunities that may be missed if we're too tired to walk.

Prayer starter: Lord, help me to care properly for my body by getting enough rest each night. Help me to awaken rejoicing, prepared to march forward doing Your will.

DAY 176

"From birth I was cast upon you; from my mother's womb you have been my God" *(Ps. 22:10).*

The Hebrew word for womb is *rechem,* which comes from the root word *racham. Racham* means "to fondle, to love, to have compassion upon, to have mercy." What a beautiful thought! My baby is growing in a place of love and compassion.

In this verse David recognizes the fact that God was with him from birth. My hope and prayer for my baby is that even from the womb she will perceive God's love and security.

Prayer starter: Father, thank You for creating my womb to be a loving, nurturing place for this baby to grow before birth. I pray for my child that she'll know even now that You are a loving, merciful God. Fill her with Your life and Your love.

DAY 177

"Return unto thy rest, O my soul; for the Lord hath dealt bountifully with thee" *(Ps. 116:7, KJV).*

Oh, I'm tired. The dryer broke on this rainy day and dirty laundry threatened to overrun my house. "Go ahead, try to ruin my day. You can't do it, soiled socks. You won't get me down, stained tablecloth." All I kept thinking as I washed clothes and hung them to dry in the musty basement was that I was going through a test. The sheets and towels conspired together to stay damp in an effort to steal my joy. "I'll get you," I threatened, running to the attic to retrieve a fan. "There! Take that!" I told the dripping laundry while turning on the fan.

The children's patience wore thin after three or four loads of laundry, so Holly and I played with paper dolls while the boys colored. When it was time for "Sesame Street," I put rice on the stove to cook, then ran back to the laundry and began to fold and stack. Benjamin didn't want to watch television, so he toddled down the stairs to help me. I must press on, but I will not press these clothes, I reasoned, smoothing the wrinkles out of a pillow case. Climbing back up the stairs with clean laundry and a sore back, I felt as if the dirty clothes had won the battle. Yes, they were clean, but I was running out of steam before they were put away.

Benjamin began to whine as a burning smell reached my nostrils. Running to the stove to check the rice, I discovered that only the bottom inch or so was completely black, ruined. The rest of the pot had that charcoal flavor that tastes so good on a hamburger but doesr't do much for brown rice.

"O Lord, I give up! How can I do one more thing?"

The baby gave me one good swift kick in the ribs, as if to say, Don't wimp out now, Mom. You're going to have to be tougher than this after I'm born!

I forgot the clean laundry and flopped down on the couch with the kids. I can find rest in the Lord. He has dealt bountifully with me. Laundry, paper dolls, Big Bird, burned rice—would I have thought a few years ago that this is how I'd spend my days?

But I can find peace, rest and satisfaction in the Lord, knowing He gives me the strength I need to do the job He's given me. I'm these kids' only mom, and I want to be the best mother to them I can possibly be.

Prayer starter: Lord, thank You for Your goodness. Thank You for Your many blessings. Father, the new life inside me is just another example of Your bounty to me. Thank You for allowing me to have Your joy, even when my tasks are mundane. Help me when I'm tired to find my rest in You.

DAY 178

"We also rejoice in our sufferings, because we know that suffering produces perseverance; perseverance, character; and character, hope" *(Rom. 5:3,4).*

I began to have heartburn a couple of nights ago. It doesn't seem to matter what I eat or when I go to bed—the burning sensation is so great that I can't sleep lying down. So I now have a bunch of pillows propping me up, a glass of milk above my head and some malted milk balls to suck so that I can try to neutralize the stomach acid.

It's easy to rejoice through this heartburn knowing that in another couple of months the root cause of this rather mild suffering is going to be born, bringing me much joy! I can overcome every complication, discomfort and obstacle, because I carry inside of me the hope and promise of new life!

Because of Jesus Christ, I can likewise rejoice in any suffering that comes my way. I look to the hope and promise of eternal life in Him and through Him. As I press on and persevere in my faith, I build character and hope.

Prayer starter: Lord, even though I get uncomfortable at times, I praise and thank You for the new life that is growing inside me. Help me to look past my own discomforts to the result of a beautiful new baby to nurture and care for.

DAY 179

"Before the mountains were born, or Thou didst give birth to the earth and the world, even from everlasting to everlasting, Thou art God" *(Ps. 90:2, NAS).*

I visited a friend in the hospital the day after she gave birth to a daughter. Sitting there in her hospital bed, listening to songs of praise, she told me that, shortly after her baby was born, she read this beautiful analogy of God's giving birth to the world.

"I never thought of God's 'giving birth' to the earth! Do you suppose He was filled with the kind of joy I have after having this beautiful baby?'' she asked.

We give birth to teeny weeny babies. The Lord gave birth to mountains, the earth—the whole universe! Yet He was God before creating the heavens and the earth. The psalm begins by stating, ''Lord, thou has been our dwelling place in all generations.'' God's kingdom is our eternal home, not the earth where we live only temporarily. That is why we must instill in our babies a thirst for the things of God!

Prayer starter: Thank You, Lord, that You understand my feelings. You gave birth, too—to the whole universe. Please bless this baby, small as he is now, to grow into a person who longs to know You, his Creator, intimately.

How do you feel? How much weight have you gained? Has God been cultivating the fruit of kindness in your life this month? What are your greatest concerns and fears? Do you have any food cravings? How is your relationship with your husband? Have you been praying for his special needs as an expectant father? What's the baby doing?

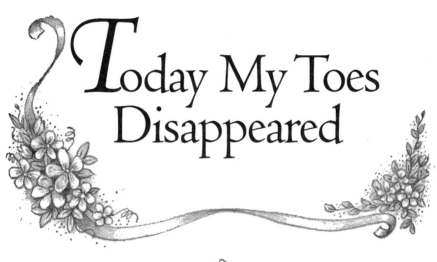

Today My Toes Disappeared

DAYS 180-209

MONTH SEVEN This month the baby will grow to around fifteen inches, weighing between two and three pounds. The vital organs are all formed, and further development will involve mostly growth. The baby's skin is wrinkled and red and covered with downy hair called "lanugo" and a creamy substance called "vernix" that protects and nourishes the skin. You will probably gain weight regularly until the last few weeks before delivery. It would be a good idea to make sure you have everything you need for the hospital trip and bringing the baby home. If you're like me, shopping becomes unpleasant with twenty to thirty pounds of extra weight to carry.

Prayer starter: Lord, help me these next few weeks to prepare for the delivery of this child. Touch my baby and form perfectly all the components of his physical development—from the tip of his head down his spine to the soles of his feet—according to Your plan.

DAY
180
"But women will be kept safe through childbirth, if they continue in faith, love and holiness with propriety" *(1 Tim. 2:15).*

Stepping on the scale this morning I can see the numbers clearly, but something's missing—my toes! I can't see my toes. I've got this huge belly, I've gained eighteen pounds, and I have three months to go!

Lord, I admit I'm scared. I'm afraid childbirth will be painful and long. I'm afraid something may go wrong. I'm concerned about my other children and my husband. I'm afraid my body will never be the same, that my stomach will forever sag and my legs will be permanently swollen and tired.

The Lord answers me through His Word: "Strengthen the feeble hands, steady the knees that give way; say to those with fearful hearts, 'Be strong, do not fear; your God will come' " (Is. 35:3,4).

Prayer starter: Lord, thank You for Your reassuring Word and deliverance from fear. Thank You for strengthening my body and giving me rest. I pray You'll continue to bless this baby this month.

DAY
181
"The fruit of the Spirit is...goodness" *(Gal. 5:22).*

The fruit of goodness starts with a thought and is followed by action. We think of good people as those who think and do good things. The fruits of kindness and goodness are closely related. Kindness is how we do good deeds.

We as humans *can* do good things without God. But it's only by His Spirit that we can do good continually. With God we even have the power to be nice to our enemies. In ourselves we are not good even if we occasionally do good things. But God, through His Son, Jesus, allows us also to partake in His goodness.

Psalm 31:19 says, "How great is your goodness, which you have stored up for those who fear you, which you bestow in the sight of men on those who take refuge in you." God has stored up His goodness to give to us. We, in turn, must sow goodness into our children.

Prayer starter: Lord, fill me with Your goodness. I desire to follow Christ's example and go about doing good to the people around me. Help me develop the fruit of goodness in my own life and to serve as an example to my child. Let his life be blessed with Your goodness.

DAY 182

"For by thee I have run through a troop; and by my God have I leaped over a wall" *(Ps. 18:29, KJV).*

Picture the vivid imagery David describes after escaping from Saul. Can't you just imagine David running supernaturally through a battalion of enemy troops, then jumping with God's strength over a wall?

My children like to sing a little chorus based on this verse: "I can run through a troop and leap over a wall. Hallelujah, hallelujah! He's my strength and my shield; He gives power to all. Hallelujah, hallelujah!"

If ever a thought enters my mind that I won't have the strength or the ability to deliver this baby, thoughts of David leaping over a wall come to mind. With God I can do anything! Can you picture yourself vaulting a wall with your big belly?

Prayer starter: Lord, thank You for the natural strength and power I have in my physical body. I know You've designed me to bear this child and that childbirth is a beautiful process ordained by You. I confess my need for spiritual strength, Lord. If my enemy, the devil, puts legions of demons before me, I can call on You for the power to run through them. If the devil throws a wall onto my path, with Your strength I can jump over that wall. Bless my baby with Your strength and power so that she, too, will be able to defeat the enemy of her soul.

DAY
183

"Did you not...clothe me with skin and flesh and knit me together with bones and sinews?" *(Job 10:10,11).*

Through all of his trials and tribulations, Job never forgot that he belonged to God. Job reminds the Lord in prayer that He created him. Job had a God-consciousness that would not go away.

When you look at your skin or see your face in the mirror, when you walk and talk, do you remember that a loving and powerful God created you in His image? Through discipline I need to make God my first priority. For me, this starts with recognizing Him as my Lord, my Creator. When my eyes first open in the morning, my heart's desire is to thank and praise God for a new day. Some days I do; some days I don't.

When Jesus taught His disciples to pray, He started by saying, "Our Father, which art in heaven." Jesus acknowledged God as Father. We must follow His example as loving children.

Prayer starter: Father, thank You for creating me in Your image. I praise and thank You that You're forming another human inside of me, clothing him with skin, knitting him with Your loving hand. Bless this baby as he grows and breathe into him a spirit that is God-conscious.

DAY
184

"So ought men to love their wives as their own bodies. He that loveth his wife loveth himself" *(Eph. 5:28, KJV).*

Thumbing through the vast amount of literature available at the doctor's office, I began to read an article about avoiding the adverse effects of pregnancy on marriage. The writer states, "While some professionals maintain that pregnancy is a 'crisis' and an inevitable source of marital stress, it is also a tremendous opportunity for a couple to relate to and connect with each other in a deeper, more profound way than ever before."

Doesn't the world have a funny way of looking at things sometimes? I admit that many pregnancies are considered 'crisis' situations, but pregnancies that are planned in a healthy, loving marriage relationship are not crises. I understand that stress can result from both happy and sad events, but this article makes pregnancy seem like a disease or mental illness. Written by a marriage therapist, example after example was given of men and women full of tension and anxiety with pregnancy-related concerns. These concerns ranged from a lack of interest in sex to fears that wives would no longer love their husbands after the baby is born, or there may be tension caused by men feeling "left out" of the pregnancy experience.

One solution the therapist gave made sense to me. "Continue communicating," he urged. Be open and honest with one another about your feelings. Another solution I see for marriage-related tension is for the wife to welcome her husband's suggestions and participation—from choosing maternity clothes and strollers to childbirth classes, visits to the doctor and meal planning. You're both going to become parents!

Most of all—and this may sound as if it is from a selfish woman's point of view but it is, in fact, from the Bible—"Husbands, love your wives..." (Eph. 5:25). Tell her you love her. Show her you love her. If she craves Chinese food, surprise her with some Moo Goo Gai Pan tonight. If she likes her back rubbed, offer to rub her back. Love her as you love your own body. Believe me, she will respond.

Now, ladies, give this book to your husbands and say, "Oh, honey, would you read me today's devotional from that wonderful book I'm reading, please. I'm on day 184."

Prayer starter: Lord, bless my marriage and help me to be the wife You want me to be. Help me to be lovable, so that it's easy for my husband to love me. Help me to return his love with fervor and passion. Guard our marriage from the attacks of the enemy. Let this baby bring a joy, strength and stability to our family.

DAY 185

"And you, my child, will be called a prophet of the Most High; for you will go on before the Lord to prepare the way for him, to give his people the knowledge of salvation through the forgiveness of their sins" *(Luke 1:76).*

John the Baptist's father, Zacharias, prophesied these words over his newborn son, declaring the Word of the Lord to the baby. What a precious sight! How exciting it must have been for Elizabeth, after the miraculous conception, pregnancy and delivery, to see her husband praising God and confirming the mission for their little son. This story gives me extra incentive to pray for my husband, so that together we will seek God's direction for our children.

John the Baptist's life and mission also serve as a reminder, woven throughout the Bible, that demonstrates a truth which comforts me in the latter days of pregnancy. Before God moves, He prepares the way. Trials and troubles need not be despised. For the chaos the world was in when John began preaching his message of repentance was only the labor pains that preceded the mission of Jesus. Subsequently, the Savior had to suffer the pain of the cross to give birth to His church.

Prayer starter: Lord, I pray that You will reveal to my husband and me a glimpse of the plan You have for this child. Help us to nurture him and train him in the way he should go. We rejoice in the trials that these latter days of pregnancy bring, knowing that we can look forward to a newborn soon.

DAY 186

"Discipline your son, and he will give you peace; he will bring delight to your soul" *(Prov. 29:17).*

Strolling with the children in a park near our house, we come across an enthusiastic puppy wearing a red bandanna, learning to play catch with a frisbee.

The frisbee soars; the puppy leaps, catching it gracefully between his teeth. He returns proudly to his master for pats and praise. The scene is repeated over and over again.

Then suddenly, the puppy spies a group of kids playing nearby with another frisbee. In a flash, he intercepts a pass, shaking his head back and forth while playfully holding the frisbee. The kids think it's great and chase after him.

Then the master sternly calls, "COME!" The party's over. The poor puppy's reproofed verbally then whacked with a newspaper.

He droops his shaggy head in shame.

I feel sad for the dog. So do the kids who ease their game away from the dog and his master. Who likes discipline? Not me. I don't enjoy giving or receiving it. But God requires us as parents to discipline our children. This discipline sometimes means praising them for acceptable behavior and punishing them for unacceptable behavior. The Bible says several times that obedience is better than sacrifice. Ask any mother who's been given peace offerings and gifts when all she really wants is love, respect and obedience.

The shaggy puppy gets a hug and a pat on his furry head. His owner shouts, "Catch!" The frisbee sails, and the dog makes another dramatic mid-air catch. He doesn't even glance at, let alone show off for, the kids who have gathered again to watch. Training goes on and someday soon this puppy will be a well-behaved dog.

Our children are much more complex and challenging than puppies. To "train them in the way they should go" we need God's help and guidance.

Prayer starter: Lord, continue to train and discipline me to be the parent You want me to be. Give my baby a teachable spirit and mind so that I'll be able to train him up in the way he should go, so that when he is old he will not turn from it. Let this child bring us peace and delight.

DAY
187
"He commanded our forefathers to teach their children, so the next generation would know them, even the children yet to be born, and they in turn would tell their children. Then they would put their trust in God and would not forget his deeds but would keep his commands" *(Ps. 78:5-7).*

While visiting my friend who is pregnant with her eighth child, the other children, three girls and four boys, discussed the merits of whether it's better to be male or female.

"Boys are weird," said one of the girls. "They hit each other and laugh about it and think it's fun to see who can burp the loudest."

"Girls don't know how to have fun," one of the boys replied, grabbing one of his brothers by the neck and capturing him in a headlock until he begged for mercy.

Boy or girl, this child is exactly what God wants it to be. My instructions are to love, nurture and teach this baby, male or female, the ways of the Lord. That teaching must be so deep and solid that it will provide the basis for my baby to teach his or her children someday.

Prayer starter: Father, give me and my husband the knowledge and discernment we need to teach our child all about You. I pray You'll bless him with wisdom and good judgment, so that he retains and utilizes the lessons he learns. Bless him and prepare him to pass on the knowledge he learns to succeeding generations.

DAY 188

"Reckless words pierce like a sword, but the tongue of the wise brings healing" *(Prov. 12:18).*

A friend called me today and repeated some very unkind words another friend said about me. "If what he said isn't true, or even if it is, I don't think he should be talking about you this way," my friend said. "You ought to confront him, because I'm not the only one he said this to."

I felt terrible, as if someone punched me in the stomach. Not only was I the subject of some stupid rumors, but a friend was spreading the lies. I pouted and stewed for a while then prayed, "Lord, You know how this bothers me. What should I do?" I didn't hear an audible voice, but I felt the Lord was saying to me, "Forget it."

Later, when Thom came home, I told him the story and asked his advice. He said very audibly, "Forget it. Sounds like a bunch of second-hand garbage to me. You'll know soon enough if it's true or not. Remember what you always tell me: whatever's not nice, whatever's stupid, and so on, keep your mind off of these things."

I forgot it and wouldn't have remembered the incident if it weren't for wanting to write it down. The sting of nasty words was healed through wise words.

Prayer starter: Lord, help me to use my tongue only to speak the truth and bring glory and honor to You. Forgive me for saying things that are not pleasing to You. Bless my baby as his tongue grows and develops. Form it perfectly, Lord, and bless it to speak wise words that bring forth healing in the hearers.

DAY 189

"Even when I am old and gray, do not forsake me, O God, till I declare your power to the next generation, your might to all who are to come" *(Ps. 71:18).*

Thom's grandmother told me that she prays for each person in our family every day.

"What kind of things do you pray about?" I asked her, assuming she prayed about our health and protection—you know, normal prayer concerns.

I was surprised when Grandmother told me she prays for my children to find godly husbands and wives, to learn to hear from God, to be raised up as soul-winners to their generation.

Although growing old and getting a little gray, Grandmother continues her work as an ambassador for Christ. Her prayers help strengthen the faith of her children, grandchildren and great-grandchildren. Her faith declares the power and might of the Lord to her descendants.

Prayer starter: Lord, thank You for the prayer warriors that have interceded on my behalf and on behalf of this child. Even as I grow older, help me to continue to declare Your goodness and love to my children and their children. I pray this baby will grow up loving and serving You and then will raise up another generation to serve You.

DAY 190

Live joyfully with the wife whom thou lovest" *(Eccl. 9:9, KJV).*

Thom peeked in on me around 7:30 a.m. One glance and he knew I wanted more sleep, a luxury I can rarely afford with three little ones.

"Get some more rest. I'll take care of everything," he said gently.

"Thanks," I murmured sleepily, thanking the Lord for such

a wonderful husband.

The next time I opened my eyes, the clock showed 11:48. I hopped out of bed, went downstairs to the kitchen where cereal bowls sat in the sink and a note was on the counter saying: "Everyone is clothed, clean, fed and happy. I took kids to Sherrie's house after breakfast. You need to get them by three o'clock."

All I could think was how happy I was for having such a sweet and wonderful husband. I called him at work to say thanks.

You may have a great husband; you may have a more difficult husband. Whatever kind of man the father of your baby is, he needs plenty of love, encouragement and prayer.

Prayer starter: Lord, I thank You so much for my husband, the father of this child. Please bless him and let him know how much I love and appreciate him. Thank You for his sensitivity and understanding of me and my feelings at this time. Thank You that he has a desire to "live joyfully" with me, the wife he loves.

DAY 191

"This shall be written for the generations to come: and the people which shall be created shall praise the Lord" *(Ps. 102:18, KJV).*

During a meeting of church leaders, the subject of children's Sunday school curriculum arose. Various teachers discussed the merits of one company's literature over another. I sat in the back, my belly bulging, contemplating the topic of conversation but unable to concentrate.

Looking around the room, I saw a large group of adults who had come to know the Lord during a move of God's Spirit upon our land. Only two of them had known the Lord as children, and one of those two had fallen away from Him for years.

What happened to the children of the last generation that experienced great revival? Hadn't their parents raised them right, trained them in the ways of the Lord, chosen the best Sunday school curriculum for their churches? I wondered to myself.

God's Spirit seemed to impress upon me that going through the motions of religion and church business does not train up succeeding generations to serve Him. We parents *must* engage in spiritual warfare, praying for our children and our children's children, reading them the Word of God, teaching them to praise, equipping them for the battle—then our children and grandchildren will be prepared to carry on the work of the Lord.

Prayer starter: Lord, I come to You once again on behalf of the baby I'm carrying and her entire generation. Pour out Your Spirit upon them. Bless these babies. Give them ears to hear and the ability to act upon Your teaching. I receive Your promise that this child will be one the Scripture foretold and that someday soon she too will praise Your name.

DAY 192

"All they that be fat upon earth shall eat and worship...They shall come, and shall declare his righteousness unto a people that shall be born" *(Ps. 22:29,31, KJV).*

Just when I thought I had run out of inspirational thoughts from the Bible that would directly connect with my current condition, God shows me another gem. Here I am sitting in the doctor's office, waiting to be weighed, and a fat-person verse jumps out!

I am fat now. My physical body is as heavy as it's ever been, and with over two months to go, I suspect this baby's weight will be a record breaker in our family. I still enjoy eating quite a bit, but I find smaller, more frequent meals are easier to eat than big ones. The eating part in this verse relates to feasting in thanks to God. He is worthy!

I accept not only my mandate from the Lord to declare His righteousness to my unborn child. But I also want to shout from the rooftops and sing out loud to my neighbors the goodness of God and His faithfulness to me and my household!

Prayer starter: Lord, thank You for providing fat from the land for me and my unborn child. I praise and thank You for my good health and strength and pray that everything that passes through to my developing child will bring health and strength to his bones. Anoint my lips, Lord, to proclaim Your righteousness to the unborn child in my womb and to his generation.

DAY 193

"And if anyone gives a cup of cold water to one of these little ones because he is my disciple, I tell you the truth, he will certainly not lose his reward" *(Matt. 10:42).*

The amniotic sac, or bag of water, where your baby has been growing, acts as a cushion of protection and a comfortable environment for the child where the temperature remains constant. Your baby drinks and inhales this water, which contains traces of vitamins, protein, sugar and digestive enzymes. The water in the amniotic sac is constantly being replenished, so it's important for your digestive tract as well as for the baby that you drink plenty of water.

The next time you have to force yourself to drink one more glass of pure water, think of it as giving a cup of water to your little one in the name of the Lord.

Prayer starter: Lord, I pray that You'll bless the amniotic fluid that surrounds my baby. I pray that nothing harmful will enter that water and that You'll help me to remember to drink plenty of water. Help me to teach this baby by example how to bless others with cups of cold water or other good deeds that will bring glory to Your name.

DAY 194

"He who formed me in the womb to be his servant" *(Is. 49:5).*

God already views our unborn children as people He has created for a purpose. Isaiah said that from before birth he was created "to bring Jacob back to him and gather Israel to himself." Perhaps God has similar plans for your little one.

Medical science has long known that from the moment of conception, as one single cell, a person's entire genetic structure is complete. Into one tiny cell God imparts all the unique characteristics that distinguish one person from another.

The fields of psychiatry and psychology, likewise, are recognizing that prebirth experiences can influence a person's mental health. Dr. Paul Tournier, in his book *The Naming of Persons* (Harper & Row), described experiments by Dr. Jean Sarkissoff of Geneva, Switzerland, for treating cases of mutism, psychogenic autism and infantile schizophrenia. The doctor played tapes of their mothers' voices with certain frequencies eliminated, so the sound duplicated what unborn children would have heard in the womb. Gradually, the tapes were made to sound more and more like the mother's actual voice, until it was duplicated exactly.

Dr. Tournier called the results remarkable. Mute children began communicating because the desire to communicate was sparked by relating to prebirth sounds. "Yes, you expectant mothers, your unborn baby can hear your voice," Dr. Tournier writes. "What does that imply? Does it not confirm what we have already said, that that child is a person long before he is born?"

More importantly, if God views our unborn babies as people, shouldn't we? We must remember we have another human being who hears what we say and how we say it.

Prayer starter: Lord, I pray You'll give me just a glimpse of my child the way You see her. I know that she's unique and that You've created her for a purpose. Help me as a mother to mold her life in the shape that You want it to take for the purposes You have established. Let my words be words that bring life.

DAY 195

"A record of the genealogy of Jesus Christ the son of David, the son of Abraham" *(Matt. 1:1).*

If you get out your Bible and turn to the genealogy of Jesus at the beginning of Matthew, you'll see name after name of fathers and sons. There are fourteen generations from Abraham to David, fourteen from David to the exile to Babylon, and fourteen from the exile to Jesus Christ.

In all these names, only four were women:
1. Tamar had twins by her father-in-law Judah.
2. Rahab, a prostitute, married Salmon and bore Boaz.
3. Ruth was a Moabitess, not a Jew. She married Boaz and bore

Obed, the father of Jesse.

4. Mary, the mother of Jesus, was unwed.

The Bible mentions these women, I believe, for a reason. Despite incest, prostitution, an unequally yoked relationship and childbirth outside of marriage, God blessed both mother and child. Even in circumstances that seem pretty strange on the surface, God continued the lineage that would bring forth Jesus Christ, the Messiah.

What does this mean to us as expectant mothers? No matter what our background or the circumstances of our pregnancies, God loves us and can use us for His purposes. Jesus Christ redeems us from all of our sins of the past, and He can redeem the circumstances of our pregnancies, good or bad, to bring honor and glory to His name.

Prayer starter: Lord, thank You again for the child You're forming inside of me. I accept and love my unborn baby, and I find joy in knowing that You have a special plan and a special place for this child in Your kingdom. Help me encourage other expectant mothers who may look on their babies as accidents.

DAY 196

"He who fears the Lord has a secure fortress, and for his children it will be a refuge" *(Prov. 14:26).*

The day we moved into our big house was a day of hard work and joy. A dozen or so friends from church came in vans and trucks and helped with the move. All day I waddled around, driving a van and giving instructions on what went where. Midday, we broke for pizza and some fellowship. Gathered in the entry way to the house, we joined hands while our pastor prayed. In dedicating our home to the Lord, the pastor imparted a blessing of peace, love and hospitality upon the house. Holly, David and even little Benjamin understood that the new house was an answer to prayer and that it was to be a place that would bring glory to the name of the Lord.

Prayer starter: Lord, thank You for the material blessings—our clothes, food and shelter—that enable us to live day by day. I'm thankful for the baby You've given me, and I pray this child will feel secure, not only because her needs are met, but because her parents fear

You. I pray this baby will find refuge in You.

DAY 197

"When anxiety was great within me, your consolation brought joy to my soul" *(Ps. 94:19).*

I visited the doctor again today. I gained another four pounds, bringing the total to twenty. Everything else was fine. I was about to leave when the doctor mentioned that he hoped I'd try to get to the hospital sooner than I had with the last two babies. He wanted to have an IV (intravenous drip) in place before delivery. (An IV hookup is a hollow needle inserted into a vein in your hand that allows fluids to drip into your bloodstream from a bottle. It's standard "prepping" procedure in many hospitals.)

"I don't want an IV. I never had one before," I told him.

He was quite firm in reminding me that I have a fibroid tumor that could cause complications during delivery. "The IV won't get in your way but will be there if you need any emergency anesthetics," he said.

I began to worry, not so much that my baby or I would be harmed, but that I'd have a long, drawn-out, unpleasant experience in the labor room of the hospital.

"Don't worry about it now," Thom said. "When we go to the hospital, we'll just tell them you don't want an IV."

"No, I trust my doctor. He knows I don't want it, and if he thinks there's a good enough reason for me to have it, I'll listen to him."

This may seem like a picky little point to some, but I was allowing myself to get worked up about it. I'd never had an IV stuck in my hand before; I had three great deliveries. Even though they occurred in a hospital, my babies were born as naturally and pleasantly as home deliveries. I didn't want to think about having my child born into a "sick room" atmosphere.

Finally, after pouting most of the day, Thom and I talked some more and decided the only thing to do was to give all my anxiety about intravenous drips, fibroids, fear of delivery day, and every other problem I could think of to the Lord.

Prayer starter: Father, You know better than I do the fears and apprehensions I have regarding the birth of this child. I pray that You'll bless my doctor with wisdom, skill and discernment. Help me turn my anxieties over to You, finding consolation and joy in Your love and peace.

"The Lord your God is God; he is the faithful God, keeping his covenant of love to a thousand generations of those who love him and who keep his commands" (Deut. 7:9).

DAY 198

"Praise be to the God and Father of our Lord Jesus Christ, the Father of compassion and the God of all comfort, who comforts us in all our troubles, so that we can comfort those in any trouble with the comfort we ourselves have received from God" *(2 Cor. 1:3,4).*

Just when I thought this pregnancy would be smooth sailing until delivery day, the devil attacked with a leg cramp. It had to be an attack of the devil because the pain was the sharpest my body's ever felt under any circumstances. Just at dawn, I started to get a tightening cramp in my calf muscle. As I reached to massage my aching leg, the calf muscle, seemingly on its own, turned into a rock, sending shooting pain up my leg.

I sat up in bed, crying out to God and cursing the devil. Thom awoke and reminded me to elevate and straighten my leg, pulling my toes toward me. He got up, rubbed the muscle firmly, while pulling my heel down and turning my toes up. The pain subsided in a few minutes, leaving a dull aching throb.

No one knows what causes leg cramps, but they're common during the last three months of pregnancy. Some say a shortage of calcium, while others say too much calcium, causes leg cramps. Fatigue, poor circulation, tension and not enough salt are also speculated as causes. Whatever the reason, there are things you can do to prevent the cramps. Get plenty of rest. Before bed, stretch your calf muscle with the help of a friend the way I described Thom's helping me. Once the cramp starts coming, turn your toes immediately toward you. Never point them down. Then pray, because through our pain and troubles God has compassion upon us and His comfort can soothe us.

Prayer starter: Lord, give me wisdom to know how I can avoid leg cramps and any other physical discomfort the devil would use to rob me of my joy and strength. I pray that, through any pain or problems that may come my way, You will have compassion on me, protecting my baby and giving us Your comfort.

DAY
199 "Generations come and generations go..." *(Eccl. 1:4).*

Sitting in a crowded shopping mall, I waited to meet Thom and the children. As I sat, I engaged in one of my favorite pastimes: people-watching. Dozens and dozens of characters with varying shapes, colors, ages and sizes strolled by, neither noticing nor caring that a little fat woman was watching. As I stared at the people, I recalled a strange statement my doctor once made to me. Pointing out that childbirth is a very natural, common, unfearful event, he said, "Look at the people walking all over the earth. Each one of them was born."

Why do I think of myself as different from everyone else? Why are my life and my baby's life so important and unique? Don't the generations just come and go, come and go? People are born; people die.

Yet even as I pondered these thoughts, I remembered the words of Isaiah: "Before I was born the Lord called me; from my birth he has made mention of my name" (Is. 49:1). Every person is unique, born with a purpose. God calls His creation to fellowship with Him. He is building His church as a glorious bride for Christ. I have a special place in that church. God has a job description that only my unique characteristics can fill.

Up the escalator came Thom with Holly and David beside him and Benjamin on his shoulders. When they spotted me, I saw four special faces light up with joy. God reminded me that the most important job I have is to minister to my family. I'm Thom's only wife and my children's only mother.

Prayer starter: Lord, thank You for creating me for a purpose. Thank You for the institution of the family and for the special role each person plays in the family. Bless the baby I'm carrying and guide him to know the unique task You have for him and for him alone.

DAY 200

"The wife's body does not belong to her alone but also to her husband. In the same way, the husband's body does not belong to him alone but also to his wife" *(1 Cor. 7:4).*

"Honey, this body we share has a very sore back, and you're the only one between the two of us who can reach where it hurts." Give your husband a scriptural plea for a back rub, and surely you won't be turned down. Hand him some liniment or lotion and he might be persuaded to rub aching feet, sore ankles and your stretching belly, too.

Likewise, you need to ask him if his body, which you co-own, needs loving attention. We pregnant women tend to get pretty self-centered, forgetting that our husbands have needs, too.

Prayer starter: Lord, I thank You for my husband and for the tender, precious love You blessed us with when we became one. Help me to be the wife my husband and You want me to be. Show me how I can serve and love him.

DAY 201

"Blessed be the Lord my strength, which teacheth my hands to war, and my fingers to fight" *(Ps. 144:1, KJV).*

I've always been a peace-loving person. Yet I know in my heart I'd fight to the death for certain reasons: the protection of my children, my home, my country.

I wonder if my parents knew the meaning of Catherine Louise when they named me. Catherine means pure. Louise means warrior. I am named "the pure warrior." Through Jesus Christ, I can be both a crusading soldier and walk on feet "shod with the gospel of peace." God teaches me to use my hands and fingers as a soldier in His army.

As Thom and I try to decide what to name this baby, I think the Lord has a special purpose for him, a unique calling upon his life.

I want the name we choose to reflect that calling. Whatever the name, I hope and pray this child will use his special talents to the glory of God.

Prayer starter: Help us, Lord, as we choose the name for this baby. Show us how to raise this baby to become a crusading warrior for You. Teach him to use his fingers and hands to do Your will.

DAY 202

"Let us then approach the throne of grace with confidence, so that we may receive mercy and find grace to help us in our time of need" *(Heb. 4:16).*

Someone very close to me has expressed concern over the conception of this child. "How will you pay your bills?" she asked. "Will you be able to care properly for another baby?" I bit my tongue and halfheartedly answered, "God will provide for my needs." To the outside world, I sound confident, yet inside I churn with doubt and fear. Will "all things work together for the good"? What if this child is a cosmic accident? Yet the Word of the Lord is clear: "Never will I leave you; never will I forsake you" (Heb. 13:5). He ordained the institution of the family. He said, "Be fruitful and multiply." He will provide for our needs.

Prayer starter: Lord, thank You that through Jesus Christ I can approach Your throne with confidence. Father, I need Your help. I confess my hurts and my fears. I put my doubts into Your all-sufficient hands and trust that You will meet all of my needs according to Your riches in glory.

DAY 203

" 'Honor your father and mother'—which is the first commandment with a promise—'that it may go well with you and that you may enjoy long life on the earth' " *(Eph. 6:2,3).*

Immediately after writing, "Children, obey your parents in the Lord, for this is right," Paul reminds the Ephesians (6:1,2) to honor their parents. As we adult children continue to honor and respect our parents, our children take notice.

Thom's parents have served the Lord in full-time ministry throughout their married lives. His mother currently has a radio talk show that I listen to with my children. One day we heard Grandma on the air telling her listeners that her children did not watch television during their pre-school years; they had no television.

"Daddy didn't get to watch TV?" Holly asked.

Before having a chance to respond, Grandma explained that once the family did get a television, she carefully monitored what programs the children watched.

Holly breathed a sigh of relief, glad that her daddy hadn't been deprived of the joys of Donald Duck and Mister Rogers. But I pointed out to her that *Grandma* decided what her daddy could and could not watch. That realization not only reinforced the rule about television we have in our house, but it also underscored the fact that Daddy obeyed and honored his mom, too.

Prayer starter: Lord, bless this baby I'm carrying and help me to teach him to honor his father and mother so that he will enjoy a long life

DAY 204

"God saw all that he had made, and it was very good" *(Gen. 1:31).*

Susan knows everything. She's always right in her own eyes. She haggles and argues with everyone who bothers to question her authority. Sadly, most of her friends avoid her. Deep inside Susan admits she is miserable. She doesn't even like, let alone love, herself. She loudly gives her opinions on every subject imaginable because she needs some feeling of worth, a sense that her life has meaning.

God is the Creator of life. He created mankind in His image, then said in His Word, "It was very good." Susan's life, my life and my baby's life are *good* in God's sight. It's so important to accept and love yourself for who you are, the special person God created.

Your baby will thrive knowing he or she is loved and special.

Prayer starter: O Lord, thank You for creating me. Thank You for creating my baby. Help us to understand truly the unique, God-given features we possess and use them for Your glory.

DAY 205

"Knowing this, that the trying of your faith worketh patience. But let patience have her perfect work, that ye may be perfect and entire, wanting nothing" *(James 1:3,4, KJV).*

I took my three children to the pediatrician's office recently for checkups. While waiting in the examination room for the doctor, the children began to get boisterous and loud. As their horseplay turned to hitting one another, my nerves started to fray. "Children!" I barked gruffly in my meanest voice. "Be quiet and do NOT touch each other."

The doctor walked in. With a kind smile he examined the children, one by one, encouraging them to express themselves. The rowdiness began again. Exasperated, I tried quietly to correct them one by one. "Benjamin, don't poke David while the doctor looks in his ear. David, please sit still for the doctor. Holly, don't play on the scale."

The doctor looked at me and said, "They're not bothering me. Are they bothering you?" That shut me up pretty quickly. The doctor may or may not have been trying to correct me, but his words convicted me.

My kids weren't being bad. I didn't need to scold them. I was the one who was being impatient and short. *I* needed disciplining; they didn't.

At the end of the exam, I gave the kids a sucker. "I'm sorry for yelling at you. You weren't being bad. Mommy just was out of patience. Will you pray and ask God to give me some more patience?"

They each nodded, then turned and raced toward the car.

"Children, don't run with suckers in your mouth!" I yelled before I could stop myself.

Prayer starter: O Father, how can any person be a good parent? Teach me to know when and how to discipline my children. Give me wisdom and patience and love to raise this new baby.

DAY 206

"A good name is more desirable than great riches" *(Prov. 22:1).*

You don't hear of many people naming their babies Jezebel or Judas or Ichabod after some of the notorious Bible characters. Babies are named with pleasant words that evoke positive images and role models.

Holly was due around Christmas (she came three weeks later). We shortened her second name, Louise to Lou, so she's Holly Lou, a continual praise to God. We remind her constantly of what joy she brings to our lives.

David knows he was named for an uncle everyone loved. He thinks he's special because of that. (Of course, he is.) He also kills Goliath several times a day. He identifies with King David. His second name, Robert, is the first or second name of both his grandfathers and two remaining uncles, so he's also named for the living male members of both of our families.

Benjamin, named for my grandfather who was a powerful, successful man, means "the son of my right arm," implying that the child will give strong support to his father and his heavenly Father. When Benjamin's old enough to understand, I'll be sure to tell him that. His middle name, Joseph, is that of one of my favorite biblical characters, a man blessed by God. When you shorten and put the two together, "Ben-Joe," you get a name closely resembling one of the instruments of praise in our family, too. (Don't worry, we call him Benjamin, not Ben-Joe.)

A good name is more desirable than riches. When we name our children, we have the opportunity to provide a forum for positive reinforcement of the values we hope to see come to pass in their lives. Our children may attain good names, because they worked to fulfill the potential their names provided.

Prayer starter: Lord, what name shall we give to this baby? Confirm to my husband and me the name You want for this child. I pray in Jesus' name that You will bless this child to do Your will and to follow after You. I know, when he does that, he will have a good name in the eyes of the world and his brothers and sisters in Christ.

DAY 207

"The heavens declare the glory of God; the skies proclaim the work of his hands" *(Ps. 19:1).*

I'm sitting on my porch watching the sun set. Hot pink streaks across a royal blue background create a spectacular ending to what has been a rather ho-hum day.

Will you, baby dear, sit on some front porch somewhere in thirty years, praising God for His beautiful heavenly handiwork? Will you be a happy mother raising children in the space age or a diligent father teaching my grandchildren the ways of the Lord?

Prayer starter: Father, I thank and praise You for Your beautiful creation. Thank You for the new life that's growing inside of me. I pray that You will direct this child's future. Even now prepare a special place in the work of Your kingdom for my baby.

DAY 208

"About midnight Paul and Silas were praying and singing hymns to God..." *(Acts 16:25).*

Do you like to sing? I do. I sing in the shower and in the car with my children; I sing in church and around the house when I'm happy. Life is a musical in our household.

Even though I like to sing, I can't imagine what it must have been like for Paul and Silas, who sang praises to God after having been wrongly beaten and thrown in jail. These saints of God, who had committed no crime, didn't have their eyes on the circumstances. They looked to God with praise and thanksgiving. What happened? The walls came tumbling down! But instead of leaving the jail, happy that a miracle had set them free, Paul and Silas chose to stay and share the love of Jesus with the jailer that had held them in captivity.

When you're sad, if the world is beating you down, think about Paul and Silas and sing! God inhabits our praise, and when we take our eyes off our circumstances and worship and serve the Lord, we can indeed overcome whatever hardships we may encounter. Our joy will point a troubled world to Jesus.

Prayer starter: Lord, I want to praise You especially when life seems hard and unfair. Give me a heart to worship You, even when times are tough. Help me to be a good influence on my children who watch how I handle adversity and strife.

DAY 209

"But we proved to be gentle among you, as a nursing mother tenderly cares for her own children" *(1 Thess. 2:7, NAS).*

The image of a nursing mother is repeated throughout Scripture to describe the intimate tenderness of godly love. The nursing child is one who is satisfied, happy and confident. "Rejoice with Jerusalem and be glad for her, all you who love her," Isaiah 66:10 says. "For you will nurse and be satisfied at her comforting breasts; you will drink deeply and delight in her overflowing abundance" (v. 11).

The warm bond between mother and child that nursing provides, combined with the excellent nutrition of breast milk, should be reason enough to plan on nursing your baby. I'm thankful to be part of a societal trend back to this practice and encourage any mother-to-be to try it. "Commit to the Lord whatever you do, and your plans will succeed" (Prov. 16:3).

Prayer starter: Lord, thank You for the tender references in Your Word to the nursing child and mother. I commit my plans for providing nourishment for this baby into Your hands, knowing that with Your help I can do anything.

Are you feeling good? What have you learned this month? How much weight have you gained? Have you had food cravings? Has God been planting His goodness in your heart? Is the baby doing anything unusual? Have you had any special words of encouragement?

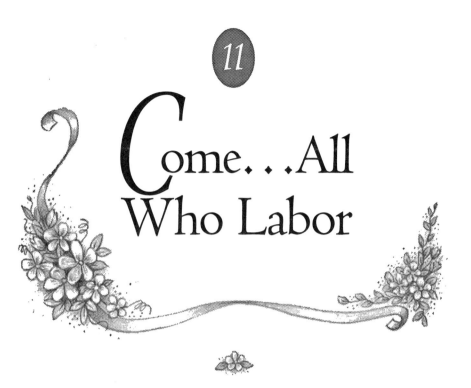

11

Come...All Who Labor

DAYS 210-239

MONTH EIGHT Your baby is almost ready! He or she weighs four to five pounds and measures between sixteen and eighteen inches. The head bones are soft and flexible which will enable them to adjust to the size of the birth canal, one of the amazing miracles of the marvelous birthing process! Fat deposits in the baby's skin start to eliminate the wrinkling. The eyes are open and fully formed and able to distinguish between light and darkness. The baby grows rapidly, putting on weight consistently until birth.

A baby born this month could very well survive but may need help breathing as the lungs are not yet fully developed. Calcium, iron and protein are especially important during these final weeks. Don't skimp on your intake of nutritious food and plenty of pure water. The brain, so crucial to all of your child's functioning, will grow quickly from now on.

This month or next, the baby will get into a head-down position for birth and drop into place. For some women (me included), this dropping of the baby transforms walking into waddling. You may begin to notice more frequent, painless "practice" contractions (called Braxton-Hicks contractions) during which you can practice breathing techniques.

Prayer starter: O Lord, as the reality of this faceless, nameless child inside of me really sinks in, prepare my heart to be the mother You want me to be. Bless this baby's continued development. Guard this little body from any harm.

DAY 210

"Come unto me, all ye that labour and are heavy laden, and I will give you rest" *(Matt. 11:28, KJV).*

The worship leader in our church has written a song with this verse as the opening lyrics. I sing this gently to myself as I lie down carefully on our waterbed. The bed makes way for my huge belly, allowing me to sleep on my side, my belly, or however I wish. This comfort is a trade-off, however, for I need a crane and forklift to get out of the waterbed. Despite the fact that I have to get up to go to the bathroom at least twice and occasionally three and four times per night, I sleep soundly. It's not quite time to labor, but I'm already heavy laden, and, indeed, the Lord gives me rest.

Prayer starter: Thank You, Father, that as Your Word says, "He giveth his beloved sleep" (Ps. 127:2, KJV). You truly are blessing me with sound, comforting sleep. I pray that You will continue to help me find both physical and spiritual rest in You as the time grows nearer and nearer for this child to be born.

DAY 211

"But the fruit of the spirit is...faithfulness" *(Gal. 5:22).*

My journey to salvation was a long, tedious process. In my early teens I thought I had examined fully the Christian faith and rejected it, thinking Christianity was illogical and inconsistent, sexist and basically irrational. In my college days I again turned away from faith in Jesus after pondering some fleeting thoughts about sacrificial love. Then, after college, the Lord Himself seemingly began to reveal His love for me.

Over and over again, people came out of the woodwork, sharing a tidbit here and a tidbit there. As a deer pants for the water in a dry place, so my soul thirsted. Not knowing it at the time, I began to search. As I studied the history of Christianity, the methods by which the Bible was written and preserved through the ages and eventually the Gospel accounts by Jesus' peers, I conceded ever so slowly some sort of acknowledgment of God's hand in the events of mankind.

I don't have the time or space to share all the exciting events that led to my conversion, but it came down to a point where I had to take a "leap of faith" to accept Jesus as Savior. I had plenty of evidence, but no one could prove anything to me. The Holy Spirit had to shed light into my heart about faith in Christ.

Paul writes to the Hebrews, "Faith is being sure of what we hope for and certain of what we do not see." By faith, I am sure that Jesus is the Son of God. The fruit of faithfulness begins as a seed at this point, the place where God's Spirit gives us faith to believe.

For faithfulness to bloom as a fruit in our lives, we must look to God and His faithfulness. In Him "love and faithfulness meet together; righteousness and peace kiss each other" (Ps. 85:10). God's faithfulness is consistent, never-changing, true to His Word, steadfast.

By faith we are saved, but through developing the fruit of faithfulness, we become steadfast, sure-footed servants and disciples of the Lord.

Prayer starter: Lord, I thank You for the measure of faith You gave me to leap past my own knowledge, which is meaningless without You, into Your knowledge. Conform me more and more into Your image each day, developing the steadfast fruit of faithfulness to trust and obey You every hour. Help me to sow seeds of faithfulness into my child, so that he will be Your faithful servant.

DAY 212

"The righteous man leads a blameless life; blessed are his children after him" *(Prov. 20:7).*

191

I read this verse to Thom at breakfast today, reminding my dear, sweet, wonderful husband that God promises blessings on our babies if he leads a blameless life. He smiled and reminded me that promises such as this apply to me also and that I bear the responsibility of leading a righteous, blameless life before God.

For my sake alone, I ought to keep my eyes on Jesus, not straying to the right or to the left. But now as I prepare to bear a child I should have extra incentive to live a righteous life. God promises blessings upon my children if *I* remain steadfast in my faith.

Prayer starter: Lord, today as I go about my chores, as I continue preparing to have this baby, remind me that it is not just for my benefit that I should lead a blameless life. When I feel the life of this little child within, remind me of Your promise of blessings upon this child, because I have been made righteous through Jesus Christ.

DAY 213

"By faith Abraham, even though he was past age—and Sarah herself was barren—was enabled to become a father because he considered him faithful who had made the promise. And so from this one man, and he as good as dead, came descendants as numerous as the stars in the sky and as countless as the sand on the seashore" *(Heb. 11:11,12).*

I wonder how Sarah and Abraham prayed as the time approached for Sarah to give birth to Isaac? Abraham had entered into a covenant with God, and through faith in God he trusted and obeyed past his circumstances until, indeed, God performed a miracle and Sarah conceived.

Toward the end of her pregnancy, surely Sarah focused not on her delivery date but on praying for those descendants that would be as numerous as the stars.

Those who love God and have been adopted into His family by receiving the salvation of Jesus Christ likewise have entered into a covenant relationship with God. We are part of Abraham and Sarah's miracle. We are among the countless children that God promised to Abraham. Therefore, we and our children can cling to the promise God gives to Father Abraham in Genesis 17:7: "I will establish my covenant as an everlasting covenant between me and you and your descendants after you.''

Prayer starter: Lord, I admit that I don't fully understand the covenant relationship that we have, but by faith in Jesus I know that I have the right to call You Father. Through that covenant, I know the covenant applies to my descendants. Bless my child and give her ears to hear Your Word, so that, like Abraham and Sarah, she will accept Your covenant by faith and nurture her children after her in the nurture and admonition of the Lord.

DAY 214

"Now to the King eternal, immortal, invisible, the only God, be honor and glory for ever and ever. Amen" *(1 Tim. 1:17).*

God lives forever. He cannot die. He is our Creator, an invisible force that designed our mortal bodies and placed them in His universe.

We are His workmanship created to bring honor and glory to His name. Our all-knowing God set into motion the miraculous process by which women give birth. In just a couple of months we will experience that process.

We have the opportunity during the childbirth experience to give glory and honor to God our Creator or to react as the world does and view a newborn baby as an evolutionary biological phenomenon. I believe that we should ''acknowledge God in all our ways,'' including childbirth. He is worthy of our praise.

When my other babies were born, a supernatural joy gave me an overwhelming, immediate desire to thank God verbally for His goodness and faithfulness. One of my friends told me that after his first son was born he and the doctor, a Christian friend, danced around the delivery room.

I'm not suggesting you preplan a special hymn of thanksgiving or any outward demonstration. But be prepared to offer your lips, body and emotions to the Holy Spirit. I believe He'll make you an instrument of praise.

Prayer starter: Lord, I praise You, because You are worthy to receive honor and glory for ever and ever. Fill me to overflowing with Your Spirit now and every day. I submit myself to the leading of Your Spirit. I pray that the birth of this child will be a witness to Your creative power and a demonstration of Your love and life.

DAY 215

"For I told him that I would judge his family forever because of the sin he knew about; his sons made themselves contemptible, and he failed to restrain them" *(1 Sam. 3:13).*

Becoming a parent is very serious business. Many times, by example and through direct commands and instructions, the Lord tells us to love and discipline our children. "The rod of correction imparts wisdom, but a child left to himself disgraces his mother" (Prov. 29:15).

God judged Eli's whole family when he did not correct his sons. Expectant parents should seek God's wisdom in child-training to avoid repeating Eli's error. Just as God, who loves us, disciplines and molds us into the people we need to become, so should we prepare to train and mold our children into the godly adults they should become.

Prayer starter: Father, teach me by Your Spirit through Your Word how to be the parent You want me to be. Bless my husband and help him as the father of this household to love and discipline our children as well. Bless this baby and give him a receptive spirit for instruction and correction that will lead to godly living.

DAY 216

"Everyone who competes in the games goes into strict training....Therefore I do not run like a man running aimlessly; I do not fight like a man beating the air. No, I beat my body and make it my slave..." *(1 Cor. 9:25-27).*

The last couple of months of pregnancy we should train as athletes preparing for a race; they exercise their bodies and eat food that will provide energy and strength. Some women endure hours and hours—even a couple of days—of labor. This is not usually as bad as it may sound, because at first the contractions can be very mild. Whether the actual time you spend in labor is fast or short, you will be experiencing a very rigorous physical workout. The uterus itself is a large and powerful muscle, and the pregnancy exercises I hope you have been performing faithfully will really make a difference on delivery day.

Don't let up on your exercises! Diligently make your body your slave; faithfully stretch your inner thighs, tighten your pelvic floor muscles, do those pelvic rocks, over and over again.

As you demonstrate your diligence in these exercises, meditate on the significance of discipline and the benefits your spiritual life could glean from regular exercise. The fruit of self-control enables us to make time for regular prayer, Bible reading and meditation, resulting in tremendous strength and growth of our spirits.

Prayer starter: Lord, teach me to train my spirit with discipline as I train my body for the birth of this child. I pray that You will pour Your Spirit out upon me, blessing me with strength and health, both physically and spiritually. Bless my baby and help me nurture her with self-control and discipline, so that as she grows into adulthood, she will be a temperate, Spirit-controlled woman.

DAY 217

"But Jesus called the children to him and said, 'Let the little children come to me, and do not hinder them, for the kingdom of God belongs to such as these' " *(Luke 18:16).*

The Greek word Luke uses in this passage for children is *brephos*, the same word he uses in the first chapter when referring to the baby in Elizabeth's womb. Obviously, Luke inspired by the Holy Spirit viewed unborn babies as unique individuals. From the moment of conception, God knows and loves each person.

As mothers getting ready to deliver our children into the world, we ought to remember that God has a unique and special purpose and place for our babies. To understand that plan, our children must know God. It is our job, our responsibility, to introduce our children to Jesus, allowing them to come to Him and never hindering them in any way.

Prayer starter: Lord, teach me to lead my baby to Jesus. Help me as a mother to show this child the way to You.

DAY 218

"God is our refuge and strength, an ever present help in trouble. Therefore we will not fear" *(Ps. 46:1,2).*

While teaching a lesson to a group of children ranging from preschool to junior high age, I asked, "What's the hardest thing going on in school for you right now?" I was amazed at how open the children were, discussing their problems that included mean teachers, threats of getting beaten up and difficulty with math, science, English and so on. I was also impressed that the children were not judgmental of one another's weaknesses. No one even laughed at my little David when he said quite seriously that the hardest thing for him at preschool was "staying in the lines" while coloring.

Whatever the problem, whether it's Pharaoh, the Red Sea, learning algebra or coloring in the lines, God is our refuge and strength. "Therefore we will not fear," I told the children, reminding myself that God will lead me through the remainder of this pregnancy, labor and delivery. I will not fear.

Prayer starter: Lord, thank You for giving me a place of refuge in You. I rely on Your strength as my body grows tired and heavy with the weight of this child that I'm carrying. I will not fear, because I know You are with me.

DAY 219

"Praise the Lord, O my soul, and forget not all his benefits" *(Ps. 103:2).*

Kathryn was in a long, drawn-out labor when her husband told her the bad news that their health insurance did not cover the baby's room in the hospital, adding a tremendous, unexpected burden to the family finances. The two of them prayed together in the labor room between contractions about the situation. Later, Kathryn asked her husband to read to her from the Bible. He turned to Psalm 103 and read the second verse, "Forget not all his benefits." They both began to laugh, knowing that God was telling them not to fret. "The Old Rugged Cross" benefits are far greater than any insurance policy. I've had babies with insurance and without insurance. I prefer having insurance. But either way we can go to the Lord with all of our needs and problems knowing He provides.

Prayer starter: Lord, I thank and praise You for Your many benefits. I place the financial worries of this pregnancy and newborn baby into Your hands, knowing You provide for all of my needs.

DAY 220

"Come near to God and he will come near to you" *(James 4:8).*

I ran around all day, first to the doctor where I got a good report, then to the office where work was piled three feet high on my desk. I picked up Holly from kindergarten, then took all three children to the grocery store. After waddling around the store, spending the monthly grocery budget on a week's worth of food, I headed home exhausted. The children quarreled over a plastic dinosaur, and I yelled, "QUIET!!!" Startled, Benjamin cried. Holly and David had their what-are-we-doing-wrong look on their faces.

"I'm sorry for yelling, kids, but Mommy's tired and irritable. When you fight it makes me mad, so stop fighting and I won't yell."

Benjamin continued to cry, so I suggested, "Let's sing a song."

"The joy of the Lord is my strength," Holly began to sing. "The joy of the Lord is my strength," David chimed in. "The joy of the Lord is my strength," I halfheartedly sang along. Over and over again we sang about the joy of the Lord, and guess what? By the time we arrived home, everyone was happy and refreshed.

While receiving the children's "help" in carrying in the groceries, I realized that in my busy day I had pretty much left out the Lord. But when I drew close to Him, through singing and prayer, He did indeed draw close to me and my family.

Prayer starter: Lord, forgive me when I take You for granted. Help me to keep my eyes on You, drawing closer and closer to You always. I pray this baby I'm carrying will have a heart to walk close to You.

DAY 221

"Those who look to him are radiant; their faces are never covered with shame" *(Ps. 34:5).*

"You look wonderful! You absolutely glow!" While we're feeling pretty frumpy, heavy laden and tired, many people insist we pregnant women "glow." I can see the glow in others, but I don't really see it in myself. Doctors attribute this glow to increased hormone levels which affect skin tone, sometimes in an attractive way and sometimes with a dulling effect. Whether your skin looks great or a little strange, it is possible to be radiant with the inner beauty that knowing Jesus brings. Add to this the excitement of having a new life growing inside of you and you may beam!

Prayer starter: Lord, thank You that I don't have to hang my head in shame. I stand before You spotless and guilt-free because of what Jesus has done for me. I pray for my baby that, however You have designed her face, it will glow with Your radiance. Bless this little face as it forms exactly according to Your plan.

DAY 222

"By the Almighty, who shall bless thee with blessings of heaven above, blessings of the deep that lieth under, blessings of the breasts, and of the womb" *(Gen. 49:25, KJV).*

After a generation or two of mostly bottle-fed babies, breast-feeding is back in style and for good reasons. Breast-feeding is simple, natural and easy for mother. There are no bottles to sterilize. Refrigerators are unnecessary. The worry of overfeeding or underfeeding baby is eliminated.

Breast milk is the best nutrition your child can receive. As long as mother is eating well-balanced meals and drinking plenty of fluids, the milk supply should be bountiful and nutritious for the baby. Breast milk provides antibodies, antiviral agents and protective bacteria that help protect the baby from disease while the immune system develops.

Some mothers never consider breast-feeding their babies for their own personal reasons. Often formula-fed infants thrive physically. But the medical community has determined that breast milk is better than formula for a number of reasons. Breast milk is easier for the baby to digest. It is thought to be helpful in the development of the baby's nerve tissues. Breast-fed babies are less prone to develop allergies, asthma and respiratory infections.

For the first few days after birth, the baby receives colostrum, a thick yellow substance that abounds with vitamins and minerals and is rich in protein. A mother who decides she must feed her baby formula should at least try to get the baby to nurse during the first several days to receive the benefits of this colostrum. Breast-feeding provides benefits for mother, too. It gives natural stimulae for the uterus to shrink into its prepregnant state, lowering the amount of blood loss. The nursing mother also develops a bond with the child and the resulting satisfaction that, as she is supplying her baby's physical needs, she also is supplying her baby's socializing needs. Best of all, breast-feeding is God's design for nurturing a newborn. His plans are the best plans.

Women whose husbands, friends and doctors encourage them in breast-feeding have more success than those who have no support. The La Leche League's *The Womanly Art of Breastfeeding* has helped me and thousands of women with questions about breast-feeding and problems that arise.

Prayer starter: Lord, You know I want my baby to receive the best nutrition available for proper growth and development. I receive Your blessings on my womb and breasts so that I'll produce milk that will cause my baby to grow strong physically. I lay at Your feet my worries and fears about whether or not I'll be able to nurse my child. I seek Your guidance and perfect will for me and for my baby's nutritional requirements.

DAY

223

"The Lord God formed the man from the dust of the ground and breathed into his nostrils the breath of life, and man became a living being" *(Gen. 2:7).*

In a normal birth, the baby's first breath outside the womb could be his hardest, because the lungs must be inflated with air. The baby must be significantly strong enough to draw in oxygen that will fill thousands of tiny sacs in the lungs. For several days breathing is irregular and more difficult than it becomes after the lungs are fully inflated and functioning normally.

Just as He breathed life into Adam, God gives our babies the natural instinct to breathe as they leave their sheltered womb and enter the world. Those first frantic cries may sound fretful, but when you hear them, rejoice! God uses the mechanics of the newborn's cries to breathe life-giving oxygen into the little lungs!

Prayer starter: Father, thank You again for the beauty of Your creation. I pray for my baby's lungs that they will be formed perfectly and will function properly at birth. I pray that these lungs will continue to operate as they're supposed to, bringing the proper amount of oxygen to my child's body at all times.

DAY

224

"I tell you the truth, if you have faith as small as a mustard seed, you can say to this mountain, 'Move from here to there,' and it will move. Nothing will be impossible for you" *(Matt. 17:20).*

With just a tiny bit of faith, you can move mountains. If you're like me, right now your number-one prayer is not to move a mountain but to insure the safe, healthy development of the baby within you.

"Whatsoever ye shall ask in prayer, believing, ye shall receive," Jesus says in Matthew 21:22 (KJV). When we pray for our unborn children's healthy, safe development and believe, we will receive our request.

Let's spend time praying for the baby right now.

Prayer starter: Lord, thank You for Your Word. I believe that with a little bit of faith, nothing will be impossible for me. You know my concerns for this baby, so I come to You in faith believing that the development of this child will be perfect. I pray for him from head to toe. Bless this baby's brain and all the developing internal organs. Bless his bones, muscles, nerves. Bless his eyes, ears, nose and mouth as they form. I ask in Jesus' name that no evil touch this baby and that You, Lord, will protect this child from harm.

DAY 225

"I waited patiently for the Lord; and he inclined unto me, and heard my cry. He brought me up also out of an horrible pit, out of the miry clay, and set my feet upon a rock, and established my goings" *(Ps. 40:1,2, KJV).*

In her book *China Cry* (New Leaf Press), Nora Lam describes the suffering she endured in a communist labor camp. Eight and a half months pregnant, she was assigned to move a mountain of coal. With two bamboo baskets attached to a poll, Nora loaded 130 pounds of coal onto her back and carried load after heavy load to a waiting truck. Her ordeal began in early May. Throughout the summer she labored in sweltering heat. She said she worked without food, water or rest.

The time came and went for the child to be born. Nora feared for her and her baby's safety and cried out to God to be delivered to freedom. God assured her that her baby was safe in her womb and gave her the peace and faith to believe the child would be born in a free land.

With God's help, Nora left the labor camp for freedom in Hong Kong in August. She had been pregnant almost a year when a chubby, healthy son, Joseph, "my child of promise," she says, was born in a free land.

I hope and pray that no expectant mother suffers the physical torture Nora Lam endured or the mental anguish of fearing for her unborn baby. But I think her story serves as an example to all of us expectant mothers to look to God and wait on Him through all of our trials and problems. He will set our feet on a solid rock and direct our path and the perfect timing for the delivery of our babies.

Prayer starter: Lord, I put my trust in You, believing that with You all things are possible. I surrender to Your lordship and know that You will cause this child to be born in Your perfect timing.

DAY 226

"A gentle answer turns away wrath, but a harsh word stirs up anger" *(Prov. 15:1).*

Rain beats at my kitchen window while tears flow into the lukewarm dishwater. I've hurt a friend; she hurt me. My ear still rings from the sting of the telephone slammed on it. Why couldn't I have said something loving, kind, gentle and understanding instead of prodding her to the point of anger? I want to call back right away and apologize so I don't have to feel so miserable, but I know she needs time to cool down.

Why am I crying so much? Why do I get irritated and defensive so quickly? That's not like me. Is it my changing hormones?

I keep bumping my belly on the front of the sink, getting my shirt wet. I wish I could wipe away all of our unkind words just as I wipe the dirt off these dishes. I think some time with the Lord and a nap will do wonders for my outlook on life.

Prayer starter: Lord, help me do what's right, even when it seems as if my emotions are out of control. Help me respond to others with gentleness and love. Forgive me for acting in an un-Christlike manner. I pray my baby will be blessed with wisdom in dealing with human relationships.

DAY 227

"How good and pleasant it is for brethren to dwell together in unity" *(Ps. 133:1, KJV).*

I had to call my friend to apologize for the stupid argument we had. Even though I still feel I'm right about the issue at hand, I can't stand the thought that we'd allow a petty discussion to get between us. Her line was busy, so I continued my project for the morning: cleaning the bassinet that Thom retrieved from the attic last night.

As I cleaned, I thought about a knockdown, drag-out, hand-to-hand combat conflict I had with one of my sisters while growing up. I can't remember if it was her orange bell bottoms or a blue tennis sweater, but I borrowed something of hers without permission. She got mad, we had words, and the next thing you know, two junior-high girls were at each other's throats. Wise Mom ended the dispute, disciplining me for helping myself to my sister's clothes and her for trying to inflict pain upon my body. In no time, we were buddies again, laughing and sharing the intimate details of our lives together. I remember how happy and proud my mother and father were because we children generally loved each other and made up after fights.

Putting the finishing touches on the now sparkling bassinet, the telephone rang.

"I've felt bad since I hung up on you yesterday," my friend said. "Forgive me. I've got such a terrible temper, and I shouldn't take it out on a pregnant lady."

"I just called you to apologize for my smart mouth," I told her. "But your line was busy."

"I got a busy signal when I first called you, too. We must have been thinking of each other at the same time!"

Just as we earthly parents like to see our children get along, our heavenly Father wants His children to love one another, bearing one another's burdens and being kind to each other. It grieves Him when we fight.

Prayer starter: Lord, thank You for my brothers and sisters in the body of Christ. Help me to be the sister You want me to be. I pray this baby will be a blessing to his brothers and sister in this family and also in the body of Christ.

DAY
228 "But we have the mind of Christ" *(1 Cor. 2:16).*

During the final eight weeks in the womb, the baby's brain grows rapidly. It's important, therefore, for mother to continue eating a well-balanced diet rich in protein, calcium and iron. With little room left to put much food into my stomach at the same time, I've been following the advice of friends who recommend eating five or six small meals rather than three big ones. In between my five or six small meals I try to munch on nutritious snacks like celery and peanut butter or apples and cheese. As I eat, I pray for my baby's developing brain. I think every mother would want her child to have the wisdom and knowledge of Solomon, so I pray this baby will be smart and excel in learning. I also hope my child uses the brain God gives, however great or small. Most of all I pray this child will have the mind of Christ, always asking, "What would Jesus do in this situation?"

Prayer starter: Lord, please bless and touch this baby's brain as it grows. I pray my child will use her brain to full capacity. Lord, most of all I want my baby to know Jesus, so that she can put on the mind of Christ as she makes decisions day to day.

DAY
229 "May your unfailing love be my comfort" *(Ps. 119:76).*

My baby constantly pokes a little hand directly into my navel. I can envision the outline of the fist. How I'd love to see and hold this little person!

From past experience, I know that it's in a baby's nature to reach out for loving contact, cuddling and warmth. These same little hands that poke my insides will soon be extended up to me for reassurance and love. Psychological researchers long ago determined that physical contact is essential for the infant's mental and physical health and development.

Just as a baby reaches to mom and dad for love and affection, so should we children of God reach to Him for comfort. His love is unfailing. He understands our hurts and problems and has His arms extended to soothe and heal us.

Prayer starter: Lord, thank You for Your unfailing love. Help me as a parent to let Your love shine through me to my child, so that he'll see not only his mother's love but the love of God as well.

DAY
230

"But they that wait upon the Lord shall renew their strength; they shall mount up with wings as eagles; they shall run, and not be weary; and they shall walk, and not faint" *(Is. 40:31, KJV).*

I've been *so* tired lately! Every day when Benjamin takes his nap, I try to lie down and sleep. But it just doesn't work. Either I stare at the ceiling worrying about all the things I'm not doing or I simply am too uncomfortable to fall asleep.

At church this week one of my friends who has four children stood up with this testimony. She said she had been weary for a long time, not just physically tired but mentally, emotionally and spiritually weary. Her husband, her children and even her church family had become sources of stress, not havens of rest. "I was close to the point of total exhaustion and despair when God quickened this word in Isaiah to me," she said. " 'Hast thou not known? hast thou not heard, that the everlasting God, the Lord, the Creator of the ends of the earth, fainteth not, neither is weary?...Even the youths shall faint and be weary, and the young men shall utterly fall' " (Is. 40:28,30, KJV).

My friend paused and explained that she had been looking to her husband and friends for strength, comfort and rest. But they were also weary. God is the One who does not grow weary or discouraged.

" 'But they that wait upon the Lord shall renew their strength...,' " she continued, but stopped when a torrent of tears interrupted her reading. She cried and cried in front of the entire congregation until she could finally conclude: "I have learned to wait upon God. He will give me the strength to fly like an eagle and run."

She sat down, looking a little embarrassed. I decided that I had to tell her how much her testimony ministered to me. After the service was over, I rushed over to her seat only to find myself in the back of a line of weary men and women who wanted to hug her and thank her for her words.

As a weary pregnant woman, I must wait upon the Lord and be renewed with His strength.

Prayer starter: O Lord, I rest in You! Thank You for giving me Your supernatural strength that builds up my body, soul and spirit. Bless my baby and help me to teach her to renew her strength in You.

DAY
231 "In all labour there is profit..." *(Prov. 14:23, KJV).*

The white paint on the walls of the room we decided should be the nursery had faded to a dingy gray. I wanted so much to have fresh paint and matching room accessories, but it seems there just won't be time to get this room looking the way I want it. Old paint needs to be scraped; the room has a lot of woodwork and high ceilings. This is a major project that will require plenty of time and money.

"Feed me and try to pay me something, and I'll come paint your nursery," an unemployed friend offered. I eagerly agreed, and he got to work. The first day he scraped and scraped, patched cracks and prepared the surface. At the end of the day, I peeked in the room, thinking I'd see something beautiful, but what I saw were splotchy walls prepared for the paint job.

"In all labor there is profit," I thought to myself, knowing that this preparation work needed to be done before the painting. The final job took four days. The result was a nursery with white walls and bright yellow woodwork trim. My accessories, varying hand-me-downs in primary colors, look lovely in the new nursery.

The great thing about having a baby is that, once you start laboring, it doesn't take days to see the profit of your work. Once those contractions start, your profit is only a few hours away from your sight! Remember this verse when you go into labor.

Prayer starter: Lord, I pray You'll be with me when my time comes to have this baby. Help me to keep my eyes on You and on the happy result of my labor.

DAY 232

"Good health to you and your household! And good health to all that is yours!" *(1 Sam. 25:6).*

During the last three months of pregnancy both mother and baby benefit from gamma globulin produced by the placenta that helps combat disease. In addition, the mother passes on to her child antibodies that protect the baby from the diseases the mother has had or has been immunized against. Nursing the baby after birth also helps the baby fight disease until the age of about six months when the baby's own immune system is sufficiently developed.

Even though I'm often tired and have a touch of heartburn every now and then, I know my body is strong. I've never had a cold or flu for the six months before or after any baby of mine was born. God's design for protecting mother and child is in operation. At the same time, I must continue to eat right, get plenty of rest, keep up my pregnancy exercises and drink plenty of water. With proper care, good health can be mine and my baby's.

Prayer starter: Lord, thank You for Your blessings of good health and strength for me and my growing child. I pray that my baby's own immune system will develop perfectly so that he'll be able to fight disease and infection.

DAY 233

"And the things you have heard me say in the presence of many witnesses entrust to reliable men who will also be qualified to teach others" *(2 Tim. 2:2).*

Paul's instructions here to Timothy represent three generations of discipleship training. Paul teaches Timothy to teach others. In this way disciples are raised up and sent out to disciple others. The church then grows geometrically.

As mothers of babies and small children, it is our responsibility to train these little ones, instilling in them from a very early age the concept that they were created in Christ to reproduce spiritually.

We should be witnesses to our friends, neighbors, relatives and the world around us. But I believe if we neglect our children's spiritual growth to minister to others, we have our priorities out of order.

Some mothers may feel their talents are not being utilized effectively if they're not being used in the spotlight. I think this is pride. God's given us a job to mold little hearts that will be the next generation of God's church. The future is in our hands. We have an awesome responsibility to disciple our own children.

Prayer starter: Lord, prepare me for discipleship training as I prepare to be a mother. Help me learn and grow in my faith so that I can teach my children to be disciples who will, in turn, train their children.

DAY 234

"Then Manoah prayed to the Lord: 'O Lord, I beg you, let the man of God you sent to us come again to teach us how to bring up the boy who is to be born'...So Manoah asked him, 'When your words are fulfilled, what is to be the rule for the boy's life and work?' " *(Judg. 13:8,12).*

Samson's father, Manoah, asked for God's help in raising his son before the baby was born. He sought God's will for his child's vocation and life. He looked to God for direction on being a good parent long before his little boy could walk or talk.

Most modern parents wait until their children have taken aptitude tests as teenagers before guiding them to one profession or another. For this child I want both my husband and me to seek God on how to raise this baby and how to direct him into the unique calling God has for him.

Prayer starter: Father, help us to be good parents, raising this child in Your admonition. Show us Your path for Him, so that we can guide him in a godly direction.

DAY 235

"For I am confident of this very thing, that He who began a good work in you will perfect it until the day of Christ Jesus" *(Phil. 1:6, NAS).*

Before I found out I was pregnant, Thom and I accepted a job to write, edit and produce a daily newspaper for a large annual Christian convention in Washington, D.C. When we discovered I was pregnant and saw that the convention was scheduled three to four weeks before my due date, we asked the Lord whether or not we should find a replacement for me. In prayer, Thom and I had a sense of peace that we should continue with our plans and that I would be fine.

My doctor confirmed that as long as I felt well there should be no trouble with my traveling the 250 miles to the convention. He even gave me the name of a trusted colleague who practiced obstetrics in Washington in case a problem arose.

My first day on the job at the convention was incredibly exciting— and tiring! We produced our first issue of the newspaper, completing the forty-page layout by the printer's deadline with just enough time to get a good night's sleep before the next day's activities began.

As I lay on the strange, hard hotel bed, I thanked the Lord for helping me accomplish more than I ever dreamed I could in one day— and for showing Thom and me the path He wanted us to walk. The good work He started in me through Jesus He performs as I follow Him. Likewise, the good work He started in me in the form of one tiny human cell He will perfect until the day of delivery. Praise God!

Prayer starter: Father, I praise and thank You for directing my path and for guiding me in ways I don't understand. I know that, as I trust in You, You'll perfect Your handiwork that grows inside of me. I'm confident that this good work You started in me will grow more and more into Your image until the day of Christ Jesus

DAY
236 "Forgive as the Lord forgave you" *(Col. 3:13).*

Glancing into the mirror, I was satisfied I looked as professional as a woman close to her ninth month of pregnancy could. Wearing a simple yet sophisticated navy blue dress with white collar and cuffs, a tape recorder over my shoulder and two cameras around my neck, I fit the role I was to play today: the convention's roving reporter.

All day, important influential men and women, including the

president of the United States, addressed the convention's attendees. I took notes and photographs, then zoomed back to the news room between sessions to write and edit stories about the day's events.

I arrived late to the last session of the evening feeling a little ragged with my blue dress rumpled and the white cuffs rolled up to my elbows. I sat on the back row in an aisle seat, taking a heavy load off my aching feet. A few minutes into the speech, the auditorium filled and even the standing room was gone. I decided to shoot some photos, so I placed my notebook, purse and tape recorder on my chair and walked about twenty feet away to get a clear shot of the stage.

As I returned to my seat, to my horror, I watched as a man removed my personal belongings, placed them under the chair then sat down. Tired, frustrated and irritated, I almost started to cry, thinking un-Christlike thoughts about a man who would put a woman's purse on the floor so that he could sit down. I approached my seat, not wanting to cause a disturbance. When the seat thief turned his head, I almost laughed out loud. I'd seen this face dozens of times on television. The man who stole my chair was a well-known Christian personality.

With his face at my belly-level, he looked up at me and apologized squeamishly. "Did I take your seat? I'm sorry," he said, without budging.

"Just let me get my things," I said softly, not wanting to disturb the people around us.

He did offer my seat back to me, but by then I had decided to go to my room for a good, self-righteous, exhausted pregnant lady's cry. I'd had it!

"I'll hold onto your things for you if it will help you," he offered. I felt like bopping him in the nose at that point but controlled myself until I got back into my room.

I wanted to indulge myself with thoughts that this man had prevented me from covering the last event of the day, but the Lord would not let me. "Bear with each other and forgive whatever grievances you may have against one another. Forgive as the Lord forgave you," Paul writes to the Colossians (3:13).

It doesn't matter that I'm nine months pregnant and tired. Christ paid the price for all of my sins through greater suffering than I'll ever know. Because I'm forgiven, I must forgive. None is perfect; even Christians make mistakes. As I forgive, I am forgiven.

Prayer starter: Lord, it seems that lately my emotions want to rise up and take control of my thoughts and actions. Help me to put on the mind of Christ and to see others the way You see them. I thank You for Your forgiveness and pray for the spiritual strength to forgive others as You've forgiven me.

DAY 237

"Therefore encourage one another and build each other up" *(1 Thess. 5:11).*

In prepared childbirth classes, husbands are told to encourage their wives during labor and delivery. In labor with our other babies, Thom has been incredibly encouraging to me, assuring me that God has everything under control and that I'm going to be fine. I'm grateful that his encouragement has been quiet and personal, directed with love to me and me alone.

I prefer his low-key approach to the cheerleading type of encouragement that obstetric nurses must be taught in school. "Come on, Cathy, you can do it!" I remember the nurses yelling with encouragement during my previous deliveries. It doesn't really bother me, but maybe I think it's a little embarrassing to have strange women jumping up and down beside me shouting, "Come on, push!" as if the delivery's some kind of wrestling match or football game. When the baby arrives, however, I feel like yelling for joy myself. That's when I really appreciate a pat on the back from my coach and the cheerleaders. "Good job" are nice words to hear.

Prayer starter: Father, I pray that my husband and those around me during labor will have words of encouragement and life that will help me do the work I'll need to do during childbirth. Help me to encourage others, including my unborn child. I pray that he will be blessed with a heart to encourage his peers toward righteousness and holy living.

DAY 238

"He who refreshes others will himself be refreshed" *(Prov. 11:25).*

Some days I feel as if I've had it with being pregnant. It's getting hard to walk. Sometimes I don't feel like enough air is getting into my lungs. My back hurts and my feet ache. When I look at my house and all of the work that's waiting for me, I want to run and hide!

It's in times like these that God inevitably brings visitors to my door needing a place to stay or a home-cooked meal. I should not have been surprised when an African couple called from the airport, explaining that Thom invited them to stay for a few days.

My thoughts instantly left me and my uncomfortable condition and began to figure out how I could pick up the clutter in the living room, make beds and prepare dinner in the half hour or so it would take for our guests to arrive. All I accomplished was finding some crackers and cheese and making some lemonade before the doorbell rang

Our guests made themselves at home, helped me make dinner and joined our family in singing some after-dinner songs. They were absolutely delightful and joyfully taught my children a song they sing in their church.

I found myself not frazzled and tired but happy and refreshed. When we get our minds off ourselves and our complaints and concentrate on blessing others, we are the ones who are blessed!

Prayer starter: Father, forgive me for my self-centered complaints. Help me to find refreshment from You by serving others. Bless my baby, and give her a heart for hospitality and strength by Your Holy Spirit to refresh others.

DAY 239

"I think it is right to refresh your memory as long as I live in the tent of this body, because I know that I will soon put it aside, as our Lord Jesus Christ has made clear to me" (2 Pet. 1:13,14).

Sitting in a rocking chair with my belly before me, I can watch as my baby's head (or is this his bottom?) rises and falls. A foot (or is this a hand?) pokes me under my bottom right rib. This child is active today!

The exciting experience of growing a baby makes me very body-conscious. Constantly I have to cast my worries about physical concerns, both mine and my baby's, on the Lord. Pokes in the belly keep me from forgetting that a child is developing right inside of me!

As exciting as the physical creation of another human being is, the body itself, the Bible tells us, is merely a temporary dwelling place for an eternal spirit person. I spend so much time thinking about the baby's health and appearance when I should be praying that this child will have a heart after God. Without the first birth, the physical life, there would be no person. But this baby's spirit must also have life—the life that comes only through reconciliation to God by Jesus Christ. My prayer as a mother is that my instruction, discipline, nurturing and love for this child will point the way to Jesus.

Prayer starter: Lord, as the spirit of this baby grows, give him a hunger and thirst for the eternal. Help me to nurture this child to serve and love You. Let him at the earliest time possible come to know the gift of life that is available to him through Your Son, Jesus.

You're coming down to the home stretch! How do you feel? Is the baby active or quiet? Has the baby dropped yet? What does your doctor say? Have you decided upon a name yet? How is the fruit of faithfulness being manifested in your life this month? Is your bag packed and ready to go to the hospital?

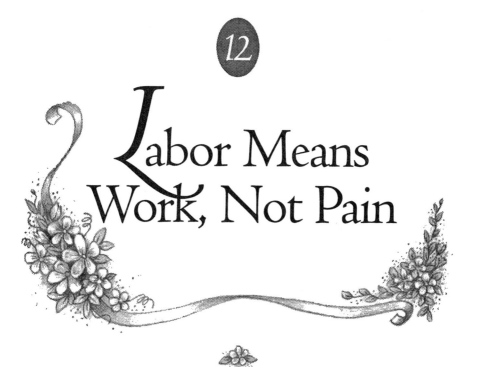

12

Labor Means Work, Not Pain

DAYS 240-266

MONTH NINE

The day of deliverance draws near! The baby this month will grow to full term, a length of around twenty inches, weighing between six and nine pounds. By the end of the month he or she will be ready for life outside the womb with lungs functioning fully. Brain cells continue to grow rapidly. The soft lanugo disappears from the skin, but the covering of vernix remains. You may feel the baby push and squirm more than kick as the womb grows more and more crowded. Make sure your suitcase is packed and that arrangements have been made for your other children if you have them.

Prayer starter: Lord, my life and my baby's life are in Your hands. Be with us these last few weeks before delivery, blessing and helping us every step along the way.

DAY
240

"Christ redeemed us from the curse of the law by becoming a curse for us...He redeemed us in order that the blessing given to Abraham might come to the Gentiles through Christ Jesus, so that by faith we might receive the promise of the Spirit" *(Gal. 3:13,14)*.

Jesus went to the cross bearing my sins, griefs and sorrows upon His back. I am free from the curse because of Him. I believe this means childbirth does not necessarily have to be painful. The curse spoken to Eve was broken through the shed blood of Jesus.

At the same time Eve received her curse, Adam was told, "Cursed is the ground...thorns and thistles shall it bring forth to thee...." Yet even before Christ, in Deuteronomy 28:4, God seemingly lifts the curse for His chosen people. He says, "Blessed shall be the fruit of thy body, and the fruit of thy ground," speaking to those who choose to obey Him. This doesn't sound like the curse of pain, thistles and thorns!

I've prayed that my childbirth experiences would not be painful. I've had three easy deliveries—one I would call painless and fun. During my first delivery there were more moments of discomfort, but most of these came when medical personnel insisted on examining me during a contraction, making relaxation nearly impossible.

For all three babies, when the actual moment of delivery was at hand, there was no pain, only exhilaration. The birth experience is truly a miraculous, joyful event. Delivering the child into the world takes work. That's what labor means, work, but not necessarily pain.

Prayer starter: Lord, I receive the atoning work that Christ did on the cross for me. I believe I've been set free from the curse; and I pray that You'll help me remember that fact when I go into labor, so that I'll rest in You and deliver this child safely, easily and painlessly.

DAY
241 "But the fruit of the Spirit is...patience" *(Gal. 5:22).*

I try to keep plenty of pizza crusts and sauce in my freezer to use when I need to make a quick meal. Today the whole gang was out running errands with me, and we arrived home later than expected. I grabbed two crusts, threw on some sauce, then chopped assorted extras like olives, peppers, onions and cheese. David, his mouth watering for anything to eat, started whining, "I'm hungry. I'm hungry."

"Please be patient. I'm making dinner as fast as I can," I told him.

A few seconds later the complaints began again. "It's taking too long! It's taking too long!" I gave him a piece of cheese.

"Please be patient, David. No one else is complaining."

I shoved the pizza in the oven and began setting the table.

"I'm hungry!" David cried.

"Honey, I've asked you to be patient. Please obey your mommy."

David grabbed my skirt with both hands, stopping me from any further movement.

"What do you mean, 'patient'?" he asked.

Laughing at myself, I sat down, pulled him to what little room was left on my lap and explained, "Patience means being happy while you wait. God tells us to be patient. See Holly and Benjamin? They're being happy while they wait for the pizza to cook. That means they're patient. Do you understand?"

He nodded. I hugged him and asked him to help me set the table, which he did happily. While getting the long-awaited pizza out of the oven, the baby danced on my tailbone.

It's taking too long, Lord. When is this baby going to be born? I caught myself thinking before my own words echoed back at me.

"Have patience; be happy while you wait."

Prayer starter: Lord, this month seems like a wonderful time to nurture the fruit of godly patience in my life. Help me by Your Spirit to be happy as I wait upon You for the perfect timing of this baby's birth. Help me also to be a patient mother to him, encouraging him to develop the fruit of patience in his life as well.

DAY
242

"A woman when she is in travail hath sorrow, because her hour is come: but as soon as she is delivered of the child, she remembereth no more the anguish, for joy that a man is born into the world" *(John 16:21, KJV)*.

Many women have pain in childbirth. Jesus recognized this when He made the comparison to His disciples with His coming death on the cross: "Ye therefore have sorrow; but I will see you again, and your heart shall rejoice...."

Women who have had tough deliveries verify the fact that the discomfort they experience is quickly forgotten after the baby arrives. Whatever kind of labor I have, I know that God is with me protecting me and my child. I know He'll be with me through the entire process. I will be full of joy when I can hold this child on the outside instead of the inside of me!

Prayer starter: Lord, I want Your perfect will to be done regarding the length of labor and delivery of this baby. You know I want an easy, fast delivery, but I know if You're with me, I can do all things.

DAY
243

"When thou liest down, thou shalt not be afraid: yea, thou shalt lie down, and thy sleep shall be sweet" *(Prov. 3:24, KJV)*.

Although I'm still a few weeks away from my due date, I feel as if the baby could come any time. I have a new fear when I try to go to sleep. I'm afraid I'll go into labor in the middle of the night, and I won't have time to care properly for my other children. Or sometimes I fear I won't have time to get to the hospital.

When these particular thoughts come into my mind, I *must* give them to the Lord. He then reassures me that I'm not having this baby alone. He is with me and will tend to me and my children. He also reminds me that my husband is prepared to care for me and the children. I can receive sweet, refreshing sleep. My fears are unfounded. I don't know *how* the circumstances of this childbirth will work, but I know *Who* is working through them.

Prayer starter: Lord, thank You for Your peaceful presence that allows me to be refreshed with sweet sleep. I confess my fears to You and trust that You will care for all the details of this baby's delivery from the beginning of labor until her first cries outside the womb.

DAY 244

"To everything there is a season, and a time to every purpose under the heaven: A time to be born..." *(Eccl. 3:1,2, KJV).*

Thumbing through my diary during the last month of my pregnancy with Holly, I see the thoughts of a more impatient me. On January 9, with my baby two weeks and two days "past due," I wrote, "I'm having contractions early in the morning. Surely, it's time for this baby to arrive, Lord?" The time for Holly to be born was on the evening of January 12. I still had a few more days to go.

Except for those who because of extenuating circumstances schedule cesarean deliveries, we expectant mothers play a waiting game during our final weeks of pregnancy. We can be happy, prayerful, patient players—or we can grumble impatiently and complain to everyone.

Keep in mind that the Lord's timing for the birth of this baby is the best timing.

Prayer starter: Father, once again I submit the cares and concerns I have regarding the birth of this child into Your hands. I trust that he will be born precisely at the time You ordained for Your purposes.

DAY 245

"I tell you the truth, unless a man is born of water and the Spirit, he cannot enter the kingdom of God. Flesh gives birth to flesh, but the Spirit gives birth to spirit" *(John 3:5,6).*

By the time the baby is ready to be born, the amniotic sac contains about a quart of water. One of the signs of labor occurs when the membrane holding the water begins to leak or suddenly breaks, releasing thirty-two ounces of fluid onto the mother. After your baby is born, and you're with a group of mothers, throw out the question, "Where were you when your water broke?" You'll probably get a number of amusing stories.

My friend Barb was getting onto a streetcar in Pittsburgh with her first baby in her arms when her water broke signaling the arrival of her second child. It was winter, and Barb was wearing boots. The water rushed into her boots, freezing her feet and adding to her overall discomfort. Despite the boots and a few more amusing details, Barb made it to the hospital and gave birth to a second son.

Susan, a pastor's wife, was singing in the choir during a Sunday morning service when her water broke. She finished the song, excused herself, then went to the hospital.

Stella was in the grocery store, horror of horrors, but a kind clerk got the manager who telephoned her husband. In a few minutes, Stella was on her way to the hospital.

I was on the delivery table, moments away from giving birth, when my water broke with the last three babies. I think John 3:5 points to the fact that we must first be born physically before we're born again of the Spirit of God.

If your water breaks in an unusual place that could be inconvenient or embarrassing, meditate on this verse and think about the fact that your baby is almost halfway to the requirements Jesus gives for entering the kingdom of heaven!

Prayer starter: Lord, I pray that You'll give me peace when the time for this baby's birth arrives, whatever circumstances I'm in. I pray that, just as surely as this child will soon be born of water, in time he'll also be born of Your Spirit.

DAY 246

"How great is the love the Father has lavished on us, that we should be called children of God! And that is what we are! The reason the world does not know us is that it did not know him. Dear friends, now we are children of God, and what we will be has not yet been made known" *(1 John 3:1,2).*

Oh, how I'd love to take just a peek and see what this baby looks like! I have boxes of baby boy clothes and at least one box of baby girl clothes. I'd like to know that everything's OK. Most of all, I want to hold this child and get to know him or her. But who this little person is has not yet been made known. I must wait until I can see this little face.

As a child of God, I am not yet what I will be when I meet the Lord, my Father, face to face. Every day I need to grow in my faith, cultivating the fruit of His Spirit in my life. I hope and pray that when I see my heavenly Father's face, He will look on me and say, "Well done, good and faithful servant."

Prayer starter: Lord, as surely as the baby inside of me will change and grow before and after birth, help me to grow in my knowledge and faith day by day. I want to become more and more like Jesus and be a godly example to my children. Even though what I will be has not yet been made known, empower me by Your Spirit to keep my eyes set on my goal: to be a pure and righteous child of God.

DAY
247
"But while they were on their way to buy the oil, the bridegroom arrived. The virgins who were ready went in with him to the wedding banquet. And the door was shut... Therefore keep watch, because you do not know the day or the hour" *(Matt. 25:10,13).*

Since Holly arrived three weeks after her due date, Thom was convinced that David would be "late" too. We were juggling a number of home improvement projects at the time. Our water pipes broke, so the plumbing was being replaced, leaving the kitchen and bathrooms torn up. We were rushing to complete the layout of our monthly newspaper, and two guests were scheduled to arrive from out of town.

David arrived three days "early" catching his father, especially, off guard. I already told you how fast David came. Thom and I awoke one morning, rushed to the hospital, and David arrived minutes after I made it to the delivery room. I came home the next day and had no kitchen and two house guests. Happily, the pipes to the bathroom had been repaired, but the floor still had a hole in it.

We laugh about it now. The women in our church brought dinner for us every day for three weeks, starting a tradition that has blessed every mother in our church who's had a baby since David's birth. The out-of-town guests have become two very close friends and brothers in the work of Christ. The experience endeared them to me in a strange sort of way.

David's birth also taught Thom and me a good lesson about being better prepared. We can laugh about broken water pipes and a new baby catching us off guard. But we won't be laughing if the Lord returns and we haven't prepared our hearts to meet Him.

Just like the arrival of a baby, no one knows the day or hour the Lord could return. We must watch and be ready, keeping our hearts pure before Him.

Prayer starter: Father, fill me with Your Holy Spirit, so that my lamp will be full and my light shining brightly for You upon the return of Your Son. Search my heart, and cleanse me of any unrighteousness by the blood of the Lamb, Christ Jesus. Prepare me also for the birth of this child—to be the mother I'll need to be to raise him or her in Your ways, Lord.

DAY 248

"Preach the Word; be prepared in season and out of season; correct, rebuke and encourage—with great patience and careful instruction" *(2 Tim. 4:2).*

Why does it seem as if everything I read in the Bible these days relates directly to me and my condition? Could it be the Holy Spirit's pouring a little more light on me than usual because I have another little person inside of me?

This verse lays out what I consider to be my job description right now:

1. *Preach the Word.* I am, first of all, a child of God. I must individually be an ambassador for Christ and share the gospel wherever I go. I am also a team with my husband. Whatever our occupations, our family's work for the Lord requires us to preach the Word to the world.

2. *Be prepared in season and out of season.* Just as I need to have

my bag packed and ready to go to the hospital any day now, I also must be prepared to do whatever God calls me to do. This means putting on the full armor of God, praying, praising, lifting His banner before me. I need to feast on His Word and be ready to take His good news to the world.

3. *Correct, rebuke and encourage—with great patience and careful instruction.* Of course, this is how a more mature Christian lovingly handles a babe in Christ. But my eyes see this instruction for me as a mother, as God's personal advice on how to raise my baby.

Prayer starter: O Lord, sow these words into my heart. With great patience and careful instruction help me to correct, rebuke and encourage this little one into godly living. Surround me with Your love and peace so that I'll be prepared in season and out of season to preach Your Word and to be the person You want me to be.

DAY
249 "He has made everything beautiful in its time" *(Eccl. 3:11).*

I don't remember seeing a newborn baby before I had Holly. Of course, I thought she was gorgeous! But when I saw other people's newborn babies I thought, "Gee, they do look a little funny."

When Benjamin was born, Thom took photographs, then dropped the roll of film off at a quick development shop so he could show the other children. David, upon seeing his cone-head brother covered with white vernix, asked, "Why does the baby have sauce all over him?" Good question.

It's fascinating to watch God's design unfold as the baby grows. The newborn is particularly beautiful to the mother through the miracle of birth. A six-month-old chubby infant that giggles and starts to crawl is adorable. What could be cuter than a two-year-old learning to sing songs all by himself? When I see a photograph of Holly on her first day of kindergarten with a toothless grin and curly hair, I wonder: How can she get more beautiful?

Everything is beautiful in its own time. As newborns in Christ, we were a little messy from the cares of the world, yet our Father in heaven and His angels rejoiced! As we grow in Christ, God loves and appreciates us at each step along the way. Eventually "when Christ, who is your life, appears, then you will also appear with him in glory," Paul writes to the Colossians. We will be made like Him, the Son, who is "the radiance of God's glory and the exact representation of his being" (Heb. 1:3).

Prayer starter: Lord, give me heavenly eyes to see my child as a beautiful creation of Yours at each stage in his physical development and as a spiritual babe who is growing more and more into the image of Jesus. Like a diamond in the rough, help me as mother to refine and polish this child through loving care to shine for You!

DAY 250

"Hear, O Lord, and answer me, for I am poor and needy. Guard my life, for I am devoted to you. You are my God; save your servant who trusts in you" *(Ps. 86:1,2).*

Fear of death in childbirth runs rampant among many expectant mothers. Statistically the fears are irrational. It's safer to have a baby than to get into an automobile these days, but very few of us fight ominous thoughts about driving a car.

If you have recurring thoughts and fears about death, capture them, confess these thoughts to God, then cast them on Him. The psalmist did this and sang, "I sought the Lord, and he answered me; he delivered me from all my fears" (Ps. 34:4).

Prayer starter: Lord, I trust that You will guard my life now, on the day of my baby's birth and until the time You call me home to be with You. I confess all my fears to You and cast them upon You. I receive Your deliverance from these fears, knowing that fear cannot dwell in Your perfect love.

DAY 251

"Wait for the Lord; be strong and take heart and wait for the Lord" *(Ps. 27:14).*

224

I'm not due for two weeks and the telephone has already begun to ring off the hook. "Are you still there?" my sister in Washington asks. "Are you still there?" Thom's cousin wants to know. "Oh, you're still there," a friend from the old neighborhood exclaims.

Yes, I'm here! I thought it would be hard to be patient, but I forgot how much my friends contribute to my impatience by saying: "Are you still there?" "Don't you feel miserable?" "I bet you wish it were all over."

I have a new answer to the questions. "Yes, I'm still here. I'm strong, taking heart, and waiting for the Lord. Yes, I'm waiting for the Lord."

I figure if the psalmist said he was waiting for the Lord twice in the same verse he had a message for us impatient people. Wait for the Lord. Wait for the Lord.

Prayer starter: Lord, as the day for delivery approaches, help me have patience and trust in You. Help me to wait upon You for all of my needs. Help me to be an encouragement for the people around me.

DAY 252

"The Lord will indeed give what is good, and our land will yield its harvest. Righteousness goes before him and prepares the way for his steps" *(Ps. 85:12,13).*

Two, three, sometimes four times a night, I drag my heavy-laden body out of bed and trudge to the bathroom. "Why, Lord, why am I unable to make it through the night without going to the bathroom? I need my sleep!"

In the early hours of the morning with my eyes half-open, the Lord speaks. There's a purpose and a reason for everything He designs. In just a short while, a newborn baby will awaken every three to four hours around the clock for feeding. God will have already prepared my body for interrupted sleep.

My two-year-old, who has not been comfortable sitting on what's left of my lap, will have less of a shock when he finds his newborn sibling at mother's breast.

My active life-style, which will need to be a little slower after the birth of my baby, actually started slowing down weeks ago as my running turned to walking and my walking into waddling.

Before giving us even a good gift, the birth of a newborn, God prepares the way. Likewise, when God gave the world the gift of life through His Son, Jesus Christ, he sent John the prophet who was one voice shouting out, "Prepare the way for the Lord."

The Lord indeed gives what is good. But before the harvest He prepares the way.

Prayer starter: Father, help me to see Your hand in everything I do. I have given my life to You and know that You want only good and perfect things for me. I praise and thank You even as I go to the bathroom at night, knowing that You're preparing me for the birth of my baby and for the harvest of the fruit of Your Spirit in my life.

DAY 253

"Charm is deceitful and beauty is vain, but a woman who fears the Lord, she shall be praised" *(Prov. 31:30, NAS).*

"Look at that funny man walking with sticks," David said loudly from the grocery cart about a man on crutches with a cast on his leg. "What's wrong with him? Was he bad?"

"It looks as if he broke his leg. That doesn't mean he's bad. That means he was hurt. But we can't tell just by looking at him why he's using crutches to walk."

David continued to stare, so I turned the corner quickly into the fruit section where I found props for an instant object lesson to explain why "you can't judge a book by its cover."

Picking up a cantaloupe and a lemon, I asked the children which one was prettier. The unanimous response was the smooth and lovely, bright yellow lemon. Which tastes better? Holly and David made sour faces just thinking about the lemon. Benjamin laughed as all agreed that the cantaloupe tasted much better. "See, you can't always tell from the outside what something's like on the inside."

Jesus tried to teach this lesson to the Pharisees with a rather strong metaphor: "Woe unto you," He says in Matthew 23:27. "For ye are like unto whited sepulchres, which indeed appear beautiful outward, but are within full of dead men's bones and of all uncleanness" (KJV).

The Lord looks on our innermost thoughts. He wants us to have pure hearts before Him. We'd all like to be pretty as peaches that are sweet on the inside, but outward appearances here on earth will make no difference to anyone in eternity.

As our bodies expand, feet and hands swell, and faces get puffy and full, remember that God is most interested in the condition of our hearts.

Prayer starter: Lord, help me to keep my priorities straight. I repent of worrying about my appearance, knowing that You care about my heart. I want to be known as a God-fearing woman because of my love and commitment to You.

DAY 254

"Let us draw near to God with a sincere heart in full assurance of faith, having our hearts sprinkled to cleanse us from a guilty conscience and having our bodies washed with pure water" *(Heb. 10:22).*

I'm lying in the bathtub on a cold, cold night. Too tired and chilly to shampoo, I piled my hair on top of my head and stuffed it into a ski cap. Cold cream is smeared all over my chapped face; my nose is red and sore from one too many blows. My big belly rises above the bubbles like a hump-backed whale.

I'm tired. I feel guilty because I did not accomplish as much as I wanted to today. I dread facing even more chores tomorrow. "What's wrong with me, Lord? Am I trying to do too much?"

The Lord's peaceful presence fills my heart. His love surrounds me. Despite my dirty hair and sore nose, I can be free of a guilty conscience. The bubbles cleansing my skin serve as a reminder that Jesus washed away all of my sin.

Even though it feels as if my baby's boxing with my rib cage and dancing on my tailbone, I know that deliverance is soon at hand. My physical discomfort is an indication that my baby is outgrowing the womb and that soon I'll hold my child outside instead of inside.

Prayer starter: Lord, thank You for the lessons You teach me daily. Thank You that through the shed blood of Jesus Christ I can be washed clean from all sin. Lord, help me to see my physical discomfort and even feelings of guilt and inadequacy as signs that precede beautiful new birth. Let this lesson sink deep into my soul, so that when I'm not pregnant, I will remember what You've taught me.

DAY 255

"Let us fix our eyes on Jesus, the author and perfecter of our faith, who for the joy set before him endured the cross, scorning its shame, and sat down at the right hand of the throne of God" *(Heb. 12:2).*

I've told you before how quick and easy my previous deliveries have been. Some say painless childbirth is a myth. I will testify to the fact that my last delivery was not only painless, it was fun. The nurse attending me was a Christian. She said, "It's OK to scream. Some people say it helps ease the pain." Right before delivery I told her that nothing hurt. Seconds after Benjamin was born, as Thom and I were praising the Lord, I told Thom, "We have to do this again. This delivery was a blast!" Ask him—he'll tell you. I had no stitches, no drugs, no pain.

Other people who have also prepared for drug-free childbirth and believe that labor means work not pain have had very difficult deliveries. I do not know why. My friend Becky, during the birth of her third child, said she meditated on Hebrews 12:2, knowing that if she fixed her eyes on Jesus she would endure labor and deliver her child. She told me, "Jesus suffered the cross for the hope of delivering the entire world from sin. I can endure labor in the hope that I'll soon be filled with joy holding my newborn baby!"

I still hope and pray that labor and the delivery of this baby will be quick and easy, but I know that God will give me the strength and endurance to do whatever I need to do.

Prayer starter: Lord, I come to You again asking that You will be with me during the birthing process, guiding and comforting me and my baby. Help me to fix my eyes on Jesus and run the course that is set before me. I pray that, just like the Hebrew women of old, I'll have the strength and fortitude to deliver this child quickly and easily. But however long or difficult the process, let me be like Jesus, looking past the suffering to the joy of the victory!

DAY 256

"I will pour out my Spirit on all people. Your sons and daughters will prophesy...Even on my servants, both men and women, I will pour out my Spirit" *(Joel 2:28,29).*

"What do you want to have, a boy or a girl?" This question is asked over and over again. Although some people have very strong preferences, I must say that I only want to have the type of child God wants me to have. I trust that this baby is the unique little person God has planned for His purposes.

It is true that Holly has been praying for a sister, but will I be upset even on her account if I'm blessed with a baby boy? No way! Whatever the sex of this baby, he or she will be trained in the ways of the Lord. This child will be taught not to put God in a box, but to allow Him free reign in his or her life. If God wants my daughter to lead an army into battle as Deborah did, I want her to be open to it. If He wants my sons to sew for a living, as Paul did when he made tents, so be it!

Male or female, this baby will be equipped to be a light to the generation now being born.

Prayer starter: Father, I pray You will pour out Your Spirit on this child, male or female. I pray this baby will have ears to hear Your Word and proclaim it to this generation. I pray this child will not be conformed to the world's way of looking at things but will be transformed daily into the image of Christ, respecting and loving all individuals, male or female.

DAY 257

"My grace is sufficient for you, for my power is made perfect in weakness" *(2 Cor. 12:9).*

Cramps, backaches, shortness of breath, interrupted sleep for trips to the bathroom—is this really God's best for me? Yet through the discomfort God's loving hand rests firmly upon me. His power is made perfect in my weakness. My sore feet remind me that I have to lean on the Lord for support. I need Him so much right now.

I thought that by becoming a mother I'd finally feel "grown up." But this experience of pregnancy and the anticipation of mothering a child forces me to come to the Lord with childlike faith, admitting my inadequacies and calling upon the power of the Lord to sustain me.

Prayer starter: Lord, I thank You and praise You for extending Your grace to me. I admit my feelings of weakness and my inadequacies. I need You, Lord, and trust that You will carry me through the end of this pregnancy and that You'll lead and guide me as a mother.

DAY 258

"The Ephraimites will become like mighty men, and their hearts will be glad as with wine. Their children will see it and be joyful; their hearts will rejoice in the Lord" *(Zech. 10:7).*

Make praise and worship part of your family's life-style. There's no need to wait until Sunday morning to sing to God. I pray that Thom and I build strong memories for our children as we sing together in the car or on the front porch swing or gather around the piano with guitars and tambourines, encouraging the children to make joyful noises with us.

When children see their parents praise God spontaneously in all circumstances, when thanksgiving with grateful hearts is a way of life, they "will see it and be joyful; their hearts will rejoice...."

Prayer starter: Father, teach me to express freely my love and appreciation to You in all circumstances. Let this baby be born into an environment known for its praise and thanksgiving unto You. Give my child a thankful heart; when he grows older, refresh his mind with memories of praising You in his youth.

DAY
259
" 'Shall I bring to the point of birth, and not give delivery?' says the Lord" *(Is. 66:9, NAS).*

Will I be pregnant forever? Will I waddle for the rest of my days with twenty extra pounds between my hips? Will my ribs always ache from the pressure of little feet squishing them?

No way! God will deliver me soon!

Just as He has been preparing me physically and mentally during these last days of pregnancy, He's also developing spiritual fruit in me that will be necessary for parenting a newborn. I've heard it said that an individual does not even understand what patience is until he or she becomes a parent. I can look at these last few days (or weeks?) as a time for God to develop patience in my life that will be used as I tend to this child.

Prayer starter: Lord, I know that You haven't brought me this far to leave me. I know that this baby will be delivered in Your perfect timing. Thank You for using this beautiful, natural process to instill patience within me. Let patience have her perfect work in me, so that, according to James 1:4, I'll be "mature and complete, not lacking anything."

DAY
260
"For God is not the author of confusion, but of peace" *(1 Cor. 14:33, KJV).*

What will we do with the children if I have to go to the hospital suddenly in the middle of the night? I know my neighbor offered to help, but do I really want to awaken her? I wonder if the hospital received my preregistration forms. Shouldn't I have received an acknowledgment? Is there film in the camera? Where is the camera?

I sometimes lie awake unable to sleep mulling over the most minute details. I *am* prepared to have this baby. My bag is packed; I'm ready to go. I must not worry about details I've already dealt with. I need to sleep, continually casting my burdens on the Lord. He does not give me a spirit of fear but of power, love and a sound mind. He gives me peace.

Prayer starter: Lord, I lay my worries and fears at Your feet again, knowing Your love casts out fear and brings peace. Help me by Your Spirit to put on the mind of Christ which assures me of a steadfast, worry-free thought life.

DAY 261

"When you pass through the waters, I will be with you" *(Is. 43:2).*

Since our birth God has been with us. Even now, as our babies are about ready to be born, God is with us and them. Many times we have seen in the Psalms, through the prophets Isaiah and Jeremiah, and through the testimonies of Mary and Elizabeth that God stays very close to mothers and their unborn children.

As your baby is delivered, the God who created that child is guiding him or her through the water of your amniotic sac into the world. "By Thee I have been sustained from my birth; Thou art He who took me from my mother's womb," says Psalm 71:6 (NAS).

Prayer starter: Lord, thank You for Your presence in my life. I know You will lead and guide this baby, even through the birth process. I place my trust in You, and I will declare Your faithfulness, telling this baby that when he passed through the waters of birth You were with him.

DAY 262

"Greater love has no one than this, that one lay down his life for his friends" *(John 15:13).*

It hurts when I walk. This baby is pounding my tailbone! It doesn't seem to matter if I wear aerobic tennis shoes with arch supports or slippers—each step puts pressure on a nerve somewhere.

I'm ashamed to complain of my discomfort when I think about the pain Jesus endured for me. His body was bruised and beaten— He was physically tortured with the crucifixion so that I could be reconciled to my heavenly Father.

He tells us that the greatest love we can display is to lay down our lives for a friend. I'm laying down my life-style and comfort temporarily for a child. I should not be a wimp. Through the example of Christ, I can have courage and an attitude of praise to be filled with joy during these last days of my pregnancy.

Prayer starter: Lord, thank You for the eternal life You gave me when Jesus laid down His life to pay for my sin. I thank You for the example I have of Your love and pray for the strength to lay down my petty complaints for the joy of bringing a child into the world.

DAY
263 "My times are in thy hand" *(Ps. 31:15a, KJV).*

Debbie recounted the last days of her second pregnancy. Her first baby, a girl, was fine and healthy, but the delivery had been difficult and resulted in her having an emergency cesarean. Her second was "overdue," and Debbie battled with anxiety.

"The days seemed endless, especially when my due date came and went," she told me. "Then God gave me this verse in Psalms, almost as a special word just for me: 'But I trusted in thee, O Lord: I said, Thou art my God. My times are in thy hand.' I got so excited! We had trusted in Him throughout the whole pregnancy, and I felt He was assuring me that the baby was fine and that everything was under control."

Prayer starter: Lord, I thank You for Your encouragement, and I receive the assurance that my times and my baby's due date are in Your hands.

DAY
264 "Now learn this lesson from the fig tree: As soon as its twigs get tender and its leaves come out, you know that summer is near. Even so, when you see all these things, you know that it is near, right at the door" *(Matt. 24:32,33).*

Expectant mothers are rarely taken by surprise with the arrival of their babies. With my other children I did not have the typical contractions that started ten minutes apart and gradually grew closer and closer together. But I made it to the hospital. Some women have a "bloody show" that signals the onset of labor. This discharge of the mucous plug could also occur a week or two before the baby's born. Rupture of the membranes usually results in the onset of labor within twelve to twenty-four hours. Pay attention to your body. Be ready to move when you recognize the signs.

Just as contractions and discomfort may signal the soon arrival of your baby, so will tribulation and world conflict precede the return of Jesus Christ. "Therefore be on the alert, for you do not know which day your Lord is coming," Matthew continues in verse 42. "For this reason you be ready too; for the Son of Man is coming at an hour when you do not think He will" (Matt. 24:44, NAS).

Prayer starter: Father, as I look for the signs of this baby's arrival and prepare myself for labor and delivery, let me also keep a watch on the times and be prepared for the return of Your Son.

DAY 265

"Therefore be clear minded and self-controlled so that you can pray" *(1 Pet.4:7).*

I'm all set to go! Before going to church tonight, I checked to make sure my bag for the hospital was ready and that I had my hospital forms and insurance information in my purse. The doctor said the baby could be born at any time, so I routinely have been putting my suitcase in the car with me when I've gone somewhere.

The actual drive to the hospital and the admission process can be frantic and confusing, or they can be peace-filled. I think the choice is yours and your husband's. There is a tendency when the day of delivery arrives to get so excited you forget things. The image of the husband speeding recklessly to the hospital is a reality for many people.

Avoid confusion! Be clear-minded and self-controlled so that you can pray. Admission to the hospital is only the beginning of the climax of these exciting past nine months. You must have a clear mind so that you can pray throughout labor and delivery.

Prayer starter: Help me to avoid confusion, Lord, by keeping my mind centered on You. Bless me with self-control so that I can pray when it's time for this baby to arrive.

DAY 266

"Sing praises to God, sing praises; sing praises to our King, sing praises" *(Ps. 47:6).*

I awoke just before dawn and noticed that my nightgown was wet. My water broke! It hadn't gushed out; it was just trickling. For some strange reason I became gripped with fear! I didn't know what to do, so I woke up Thom and told him my water had broken.

"Are you having any contractions?" he asked. When I told him I wasn't, he asked me to try to go back to sleep.

"Honey, I'm really scared. I can't go to sleep!"

Thom reached over and prayed, "Lord, we know that Cathy and this baby are totally in Your loving care that drives out all fear. I rebuke this fear in Jesus' name and pray that Your peace will fill Cathy's heart. I pray the delivery of this baby will be quick, easy and safe. Amen."

I began to meditate on Psalm 23:4: "I will fear no evil, for you are with me." I fell asleep.

While I was still asleep, Thom took the children to my friend Sherrie's house. Around 10:00 a.m., still having no contractions, I got up, took a shower and thought about calling the doctor. I had one or two very mild contractions, but I'd been having those for weeks. I got scared again, thinking the doctor would want to induce the birthing.

"O God, I don't want to be induced. If it's time for this baby to be born, please let the birth happen quickly and naturally." I went to my word processor and continued to work on these devotions. Then I curled my hair.

As I was combing out my curls and putting on makeup, Thom showed up at the door with a video camera, asking me to share beauty tips for women on their way to the hospital to have a baby. (This video turned out to be a home classic.)

I called the doctor, and he said what I knew he'd say: "Come to the hospital now."

Thom continued his video production as I got into the car and we drove to the hospital. A tape of praise music played in the background the entire time giving a nice sound track for his movie.

I was admitted into the hospital and taken to the labor room where I haggled with the nurses a little about not wanting a fetal monitor before I was examined. I still didn't feel as if I was in labor and I did not want to be strapped into a bed!

My doctor examined me after I'd been in the hospital for an hour or so. I was dilated about four centimeters, so he thought it could be hours before the baby would arrive.

I asked to be transferred to the birthing suite and within a few minutes was settled into a very pleasant room. This was about 3:30 in the afternoon. After a little while, I had an extremely intense contraction during which I tried to relax and breathe deeply and slowly. Yes, I'm really going to have a baby!

I prepared mentally for a number of contractions, but they didn't come. After about fifteen minutes I had another really powerful contraction. Then after another fifteen minutes I had a third contraction, and during this contraction I felt like pushing. I buzzed for the nurse who came scurrying into the room. A doctor followed shortly, quickly examining me and announcing, "You're over ten centimeters dilated. As soon as we're set up, you can push."

Hallelujah! I loved hearing those words!

My doctor arrived and realized there was no time to hook up the IV I didn't want. "You always get your own way, don't you?" he said good-naturedly.

On the next contraction Jeana Joy was born into the world, screaming and wiggling. When I heard the doctor say, "It's a girl!" everything inside me wanted to get up off the bed and dance and sing praises to God!

My baby was born quickly and easily! Holly's prayers for a sister were answered! No stitches! No complications with the fibroid tumor! Praise God. Thank You for this new little creation made in Your image.

Thom praised the Lord with me as Jeana, still covered with vernix, nursed vigorously and the doctors and nurses ran around doing what they do at times like this. When the baby was cleaned up and given back to me, Thom and I had a time of prayer and dedication together. Then we started to call everyone. He continued his video production, and after viewing it later I was very happy I'd decided to curl my hair and put on makeup.

Within an hour Holly, David and Benjamin came to visit their new sister. They all seemed pretty happy and excited. Grandpa Hickling, with Grandma at his side, led the family in a prayer of dedication for the new baby and welcomed her officially into the clan.

After everyone went home, I stayed up with my precious Jeana, staring at her delicate fingers and beautiful face. I thought of the day I found out I was pregnant and remembered the Lord impressed upon me that this tiny, helpless baby would be created in the image of God.

Prayer starter: Father, thank You for taking me every step along the way throughout this pregnancy. Thank You for this baby, this precious gift. Help my husband and me to be good parents. Bless this baby and help her to grow to love and serve You.

For all those who remain ladies-in-waiting after day 266, here's a great idea. Go back to the first day of the ninth month and repeat these devotions! Don't be upset or nervous. Your day will come!

For a free wallet-size card with Bible Promises for Pregnancy and information about other resources for young parents, send a stamped, self-addressed envelope to:

Cathy Hickling
P.O. Box 44148
Pittsburgh, PA 15205